ORTHODONTICS IN AN AGING SOCIETY

This volume includes the proceedings
of the Annual Symposium on Craniofacial Growth
February 19-20, 1988, Ann Arbor, Michigan

Editor
DAVID S. CARLSON

Editorial Associate
ANDREA FERRARA

This volume is supported in part by
USPHS Grant DE 03610

Monograph 22
Craniofacial Growth Series

Center for Human Growth and Development
The University of Michigan
Ann Arbor, Michigan

Publisher's Cataloging in Publication Data

Center for Human Growth and Development
Craniofacial Growth Monograph Series
Orthodontics in an aging society.
Monograph 22

ISSN 0162-7279
ISBN 0-929921-00-3 (series)
ISBN 0-929921-18-6 (volume)
Library of Congress Catalog Card Number 88-71195

SYMPOSIUM PARTICIPANTS

Speakers

W. ANDREW ACHENBAUM, Institute of Gerontology, The University of Michigan, Ann Arbor, Michigan

RICHARD C. ADELMAN, Institute of Gerontology, The University of Michigan, Ann Arbor, Michigan

ROLF G. BEHRENTS, Department of Orthodontics, The University of Tennessee, Memphis, Tennessee

JEFFREY B. HALTER, Institute of Gerontology, The University of Michigan, Ann Arbor, Michigan

BIRTE MELSEN, Department of Orthodontics, Royal Dental College, Aarhus, Denmark

WILLIAM R. PROFFIT, Department of Orthodontics, University of North Carolina, Chapel Hill, North Carolina

CHRISTIAN S. STOHLER, Department of Restorative Dentistry, School of Dentistry, The University of Michigan, Ann Arbor, Michigan

Discussion Leaders

BRIAN A. BURT, School of Public Health and School of Dentistry, The University of Michigan, Ann Arbor, Michigan

CHESTER A. DOUGLASS, Harvard School of Dental Medicine, Harvard University, Boston, Massachusetts

DONALD H. ENLOW, Department of Orthodontics, Case Western Reserve University, Cleveland, Ohio

STANLEY M. GARN, Center for Human Growth and Development and Department of Anthropology, The University of Michigan, Ann Arbor, Michigan

SOLICITED CONTRIBUTORS

URBAN HÄGG, Department of Orthodontics, University of Lund, Mälmo; Department of Anatomy, and Department of Pediatrics, Gothenburg University, Göteborg, Sweden

JOHAN KARLBERG, Department of Pediatrics, Gothenburg University, Göteborg, Sweden

ALEXANDRE G. PETROVIC, National Institute of Health and Medical Research, Strasbourg, France

JEANNE J. STUTZMANN, National Institute of Health and Medical Research, Strasbourg, France

JOHN TARANGER, Department of Pediatrics, Gothenburg University, Göteborg, Sweden

TABLE OF CONTENTS

PREFACE

Orthodontic training, both with respect to orthodontic theory and orthodontic practice, has traditionally dealt primarily with problems related to development, growth, and treatment of craniofacial disorders that occur during childhood and adolescence. Today, however, there is an increasing demand for orthodontic treatment of adult patients, patients who are beyond adolescence. These adult patients often not only manifest a greatly diminished growth potential, but they also may have malocclusions that are significantly compromised by dental diseases and the loss of teeth. Collectively, such patients present a number of problems that are rarely addressed in textbooks, orthodontic programs, and short courses. It was with these problems in mind that the 15th Annual Symposium on Craniofacial Growth, *Orthodontics in an Aging Society*, was held on February 19-20, 1988 in Ann Arbor, Michigan. This book provides the proceedings of that symposium.

The three general goals of the Symposium are also the three major goals of this book. The first goal is to provide authoritative background information about our aging society and about the aging process itself. It has become a cliché to state that there has been a significant increase in the mean age of industrialized populations, that there is a "graying" of contemporary society. To what extent is this cliché accurate? What are the factors that are operable and the trends that we can expect as time goes on? Finally, what are the ramifications of these trends for delivery of dental and medical health care? Professors Andrew Achenbaum, Richard Adelman, and Jeffrey Halter of the Institute of Gerontology of The University of Michigan and Professors Stanley Garn and Brian Burt, of The University of Michigan's Center for Human Growth & Development and School of Public Health, respectively, present extensive discussions addressing each of these areas.

The second goal of this book is to review current information about the changes in the craniofacial complex that take place in the adult, after it is assumed that most growth has been completed. It is generally assumed that there are no significant changes in the craniofacial skeleton after adulthood has been achieved. However, recent information provided by Professors Rolf Behrents of the University of Tennessee and

Donald Enlow of Case Western Reserve University indicates that significant changes, many of which may be of profound clinical significance, may occur in the craniofacial skeleton long after adulthood has been reached.

The third goal is to provide specific information concerning strategies for management of older orthodontic patients. Orthodontic treatment of patients who manifest a degenerating dentition due to periodontal disease is a particular concern in adults. Professor Birte Melsen of Aarhus University provides an excellent overview of clinical management of adult patients with compromised dentitions. A second clinical area that is becoming of increasing concern is the subject of temporomandibular disorders. Professor Christian Stohler of The University of Michigan provides a fresh review of the available epidemiological data as well as original research data on this subject as it relates to both young adults and the elderly. Professor William Proffit of the University of North Carolina provides an overview of the significance of previous and current trends in the biology of aging, population dynamics, and health care delivery for treatment of craniofacial disorders in general and for orthodontics in particular.

Finally, Professor Urban Hägg from the University of Lund provides the most current information on the developmental transition from adolescence to adulthood in males, and Professor Jeanne Stutzmann of the University of Strasbourg describes recent experimental research on human subjects that deals with the biological mechanisms of tooth movement and alveolar bone remodeling in adults.

The 15th Annual Symposium on Craniofacial Growth, as in the past, was co-sponsored by the Center for Human Growth & Development and the School of Dentistry of The University of Michigan and honored Professor Robert E. Moyers, Professor of Dentistry and Fellow of the Center for Human Growth & Development. Financial support for the Symposium was solely through the revenues obtained through the sale of previously published volumes in the Craniofacial Growth Monograph Series of the Center for Human Growth and Development and from donations to the "Friends of the Symposium" fund.

FRIENDS OF THE MOYERS SYMPOSIUM

Patrons

Dr. Roy D. McAnnally
Anonymous

Friends

Dr. Rolf & Mrs. Eileen Behrents
Dr. Patrick A. Bernardi
Dr. Donald Bookman
Dr. Charles R. Cushing
Dr. Jos Dibbets
Dr. R.W. Faith
Dr. Robert Fisher
Dr. Ronald Gardin
Dr. Lee W. Graber
Dr. Gary E. Hall
Dr. K. Michael Hayes
Dr. Stephen Hershey
Dr. Richard Herz
Dr. Robert J. Isaacson
J.C.O., Inc.
Dr. Joseph R. Jarabak
Dr. W. John Jenkins
Dr. Lysle Johnston
Dr. Henry Kaplan
Dr. George H. Kho
Dr. Wendell C. Kitchin
Dr. Ruth Kukulski
Dr. James F. Laidlaw
Dr. Joseph Lehman
Dr. Edward E. Linsel, Jr.
Dr. Herbert Lippitz
Dr. Colin Mayers
Dr. Earl McWherter
Dr. Angelos Metaxas
Dr. Peter N. Neuman
Oregon Orthodontic Alumni
Dr. William A. Patchak
Dr. Elmo W. Penley
Dr. Norman H. Pokley
Dr. Verne M. Primack
Dr. Galen Quinn
Dr. O.H. Rigsbee
Dr. Sergius A. Rinaldi
Dr. Lawrence Rosenberg
Dr. Sheldon Rosenstein
Dr. Arnold Rosenthal
Dr. Robert Shaye
Dr. Ralph H. Smith
Dr. Dean B. Sommerfield
Dr. James P. Stenger
Dr. Jerome Weiss
Dr. Billy West
Dr. Daryl E. Williams
Dr. Walter Winter

Donors

Dr. Alan R. Dutkin
Dr. Anna C. Ettinger
Dr. Ahmed A. Uthman
Dr. Ted Wachna

THE AGING SOCIETY

W. Andrew Achenbaum

As an historian who is frequently asked to speak at gatherings of nonhistorians, I often have the feeling that I mainly am expected to share a few amusing anecdotes from that treasure-trove known as "historical data." Then, having said my piece as humorously and inspiringly as possible, I sense that I am to step aside quickly so that the serious participants can get down to the important business at hand.

Such is the crisis of confidence in the historians' ranks. With Christopher Lasch (1979) we deplore the pervasive American "culture of narcissism" that makes seeking lessons from our past a tedious, irrelevant business for most of our non-historian colleagues. Or we admit among ourselves that we can't be bothered accepting invitations to multidisciplinary ventures—unless the hosts focus on an issue or highlight a methodology that will advance our own parochial predilections and/or impress our peers. Sometimes historians are so oblivious to the possibility that other researchers are pursuing the very questions that engage us, albeit by using different techniques and seemingly orthogonal procedures, that we miss genuinely exciting possibilities for our own intellectual growth.

The general goals of this paper are to provide a perspective and to highlight those factors that are worth noting about human life in an aging society. In this respect, it should be noted at the outset that historians do not just talk about the past; historians investigate continuities and changes over time. They are interested in describing and explaining how ordinary people, politicians, professionals, partisans, philanderers, polyglots, presidents, parents, priests, and plutocrats (among other personages) attempt to cope with ever-changing circumstances. Historians study conditions over which they often had, have, or will have little control.

In order to achieve these goals, the first half of this paper will consider trends that pertain to the novel notion of an "aging society." My thesis, quite bluntly, is that the inexorable aging of America's population will affect every institution in our society and the ways people live in the twenty-first century.

Declining fertility rates, gains in adult longevity, and the size of the baby-boom cohort have already necessitated changes in health-care delivery, educational programs, and pension systems. These demographic factors will influence how we choose to invest in youth and minorities and to capitalize on the human resource potentials of mature men and women. They require us to think anew about the creative tensions between protecting individual rights and promoting collective responsibilities. Viewing the United States (and most other advanced-industrial countries) as an aging society raises fundamental questions about citizenship and mutual dependence, domestically and across national boundaries. Sooner or later, it will demand bold policy initiatives in both the public and private sectors.

The second half of this paper will deal with a pattern of thought and behavior which is not novel. Indeed, the fact that we hew to outmoded styles and conventions may put us at a disadvantage as we seek to get a handle on societal aging. Quite simply, few academic researchers take "age" seriously. Biomedical investigators, behavioral and social scientists, and humanists alike fail to distinguish among age, aging, and the aged. They confound societal and individual aging. Age is used in the scholarly literature as both an independent and dependent variable (Maddox and Campbell, 1985; Achenbaum, 1987). If university-based researchers and teachers want to grapple effectively with the promises and paradoxes that inhere in novel circumstances, then they will need to transform the prevailing manner of going about their business.

Tracing the history of the Institute of Gerontology at The University of Michigan can provide a useful illustration of continuities and changes in how researchers think about "age." During the past half-century, research at the Institute of Gerontology has become more scientific in its self-representations. Paradoxically, however, it is not at all self-evident that gerontology can ever flourish as a comprehensive science, there or elsewhere. Hence, determining the tradeoffs of fulfilling discipline-specific obligations at the expense of engaging in interdisciplinary ventures to do basic or applied research is an acute matter before all of us. For example, because of demographic changes related to aging, orthodontists and other oral health specialists have a real stake in changing the status quo. To adapt to an aging society, an expertise will be needed that is not readily available in the university, which remains the font of most professional innovation (Haskell, 1984).

THREE NEW TRENDS IN SOCIETAL AGING

Demographic Projections

The first trend related to societal aging worth noting is that in the decades to come there will be proportionately fewer children and greatly increased numbers of middle-aged and older people in the United States. This single demographic factor will alter nearly every aspect of life, including who gets braces, who works in the office, and who pays for orthodontics. It is important, therefore, to appreciate the novel features of this phenomenon.

The aging of America per se is not new: it results primarily from two centuries of declining birth rates. Whereas in 1790 half of the population was under the age of 16, this percent has now receded to about 22 percent, and is expected to continue to decline. This long-term trend, however, lately has become far more noticeable and salient, partly because of significant gains in adult longevity since World War II (U.S. Bureau of Census, 1984). The proportion of our population over the age of 65 has risen from eight percent to 12 percent during the past 35 years and is still growing. The old-old age group is the fastest growing segment; demographers predict that there will be some 16 million Americans over the age of 85 by the middle of the next century. The baby-boom generation, which gave new meaning to "youth" in the 1960s and is now beginning to alter our images of "middle age," will constitute an incredible demographic bulge in "the third quarter of life": the years between 50 and 75 (Jones, 1980).

Hence what is striking about societal aging nowadays is the rapid pace at which changes in the relative proportions of young, middle-aged and elderly citizens are transforming our demographic structure. The population triangle that once existed in most developed nations—with many children at the base and a relatively small number of older men and women at the top—is giving way to a situation in which a very substantial and diverse number of elders vies for goods and services with youths and baby-boomers, with each group making their own, quite specific, societal demands. We are at the threshold of a societal revolution that may have consequences as significant as those wrought earlier this century by technological changes in transportation and communication. It already has begun to affect political claims across age lines (Longman, 1987).

A major ramification of these demographic transformations is that people of all ages are longer-lived than ever before. A child born in the United States in 1790 had no greater and no lesser a probability of celebrating her or his first birthday than a child born 180 years later has of attaining age 70 (Demos, 1986). What this reminds us, of course, is that there have been remarkable gains in infant and child mortality rates, thanks to improvements in public health, medical technology and practice, and patient self-care (Starr, 1982). Nor has the 26-year extension of life expectancy since 1900 simply resulted from improvements at the younger end of the life course. In 1940, men and women who were aged 65 could not expect to live much longer than their forebears at the end of the American Revolution—about 6 to 8 years, with women, on the average, living about 2.2 years longer than men. By 1983, the older were living longer—men could expect to live an additional 14.2 years, and women another 18.6 years (Riley and Riley, 1986)—and the gender differential had broadened.

Who Will Shape Society?

This suggests a second trend: an aging society, demographically and socio-economically, will increasingly be shaped by more and more women who are coping and adapting to changing roles at different moments in their lives. Demographically, the feminization of the population structure is quite remarkable (Achenbaum, 1978; Rossi, 1985). Between 1900 and 1930, only a slightly greater proportion of all women than men were over 65 years old. By 1970, in contrast, 8.5% of all men, compared to 11.2% of all women, were at least 65 years old. This trend is expected to continue over time. It is also worth noting that it was not until the 1940 census that there were actually more older females than older males. (This is because, historically, more women died in childbirth than men died of wounds or poor medical attention on the battlefield.) This shift, too, has become more apparent since World War II. In 1986 there was a sex ratio of 147 women over 65 years of age for every 100 men in that age group. The sex ratio increased with age, rising from 121 women per 100 men for the 65- to 69-year old group to a high of 253 for persons 85 and over. Since a slightly greater number of baby boys are born than are baby girls, there surely is fodder here for a discussion of the comparative strengths of the sexes!

Perhaps more significant than demographic changes in the balance between the sexes have been the newsworthy arrangements and shifts in attitudes taking place due to the subtle revolution in the marketplace and in the bedroom. Women have always worked, to be sure, but for the first time more than half of them are being compensated for what they do. More than 50% of all married and single women, more than 50% of those who have raised their children, and more than 50% of those with children under five, are in the marketplace. The Equal Pay Act (1963) and the 1964-65 Civil Rights legislation made it illegal to discriminate on the basis of sex. Women nevertheless encounter sex discrimination in the job market; they remain clustered in a finite number of traditionally "women's" jobs. The situation is changing—a third of all students in dental school (to pick a pertinent example) are women—but slowly (Brown and Pechman, 1987). Job discrimination often translates into pay discrimination: women now earn roughly 74 cents for every one dollar men earn—although this figure is up from 69 cents two decades ago, equality remains an elusive dream for women.

Still, having more income at their disposal has apparently enabled women to make the tough choices between work and family in ways they presumably find preferable, or at least more tolerable, than conditions their mothers found. Women remain primary care-givers. But they have more options for back-up support, including, sometimes, the decision to delay or postpone indefinitely the responsibility of parenting. With declining fertility, the number of children a woman must nurture has declined. The likelihood that she will be attending to her aging parent(s) has concurrently increased, particularly in the twentieth century. This gives women, on one hand, more opportunity for lasting same-sex relationships with kin than has ever existed before. On the other hand, it creates fresh sources of marital disputes, which partly accounts for the fact that half of all first marriages are dissolved within seven years (Friedan, 1981; Hagestad, 1985).

Age and Human Experience

The widening gap in numbers between old(er) males and females points to a third trend: the range of human experiences from womb to tomb will become ever more variegated. The social meanings of age are changing as the boundaries between life periods are blurring (Neugarten and Neugarten, 1986). Some women have their first child at the age of 14. Others wait until they are in their late thirties. This produces first-time grandmothers who range in age from 35 to 75. Similarly, with increasing tracking and specialization in our educational system, some individuals enter the job market in low-skilled positions upon graduating from high school, others do not finish their doctoral studies or professional training until they are around thirty, and still others are returning to school after age forty to prepare for a second or third career in mid-life. Such fluidity in social roles and age norms has led to a situation in which people are paradoxically more anxious and more confident because they no longer slavishly conform to rules (Veroff *et al.*, 1981; Sorenson *et al.*, 1986).

Reinforcing these trends is a host of new developments that contribute to the diversity of experiences in the United States. The Hispanic citizenry of our population is growing rapidly; it is not at all clear that Chicanos or Latinos will conform to the familial or political patterns of accommodation and adaptation as immigrants from southern and eastern Europe did earlier in the century (Torres-Gil, 1986). Similarly, we now have a clearer understanding of the ecological, ideological, economic, and structural problems that have exacerbated the plight of the underclass in the nation's inner cities (Wilson, 1987). This, coupled with the uncertainty of the nation's economy and competitive standing in the international arena (Calleo, 1982), all ensure that the future holds very different things for various segments of our population.

Implications for Oral Health Specialists

In light of such diversity, what are the ramifications of an aging society for orthodontists and other oral health specialists? Clearly, emphasis should focus on the physical capacities, human resource talents, and needs of men and women who are (or shortly will be) in the "third quarter of life." Roughly a fifth of the population is between the ages of 50 and 75 years of age: by 2010, about one out of every three Americans will be in this age range. I suspect that people at the lower end of this age range will seek orthodontics. As a profession, orthodontists will grow older; so will their staffs. In tapping the potential of a large number of citizens over fifty years of age, the issue of their continued productivity (or lack thereof) will undoubtedly be important, and have a major impact on the overall state of the economy. Rather than continuing to encourage people to "retire" from contributing their services at a given age, ways should be devised to ensure that the "third quarter of life" is a period of renewal, which awakens new interests and opens up fresh possibilities (Pifer, 1986).

THE THIRD QUARTER OF LIFE

It is important to note how little is known about continuities and changes in the biological, behavioral, and social processes of men and women over 40, prior to the onset of old age. "The third quarter of life"—whatever its chronological borders (and it may lack precise boundaries)—is at present largely unexplored territory. Since the 1930s, we have become accustomed to segmenting the adult life course in a fairly rigid way: majority at age 21, middle age at 40, work or career until the seventh decade, old age at 65, decline soon thereafter. In many ways this has been very convenient. Because of the familiarity of this pattern, there has been some resistance to defining the life course differently. As Henry Nash Smith once said, all of us are, to some extent, creatures of a historical tradition—a particular social structure, conditioned by our family and our own personal circumstances. These contextual factors create a screen through which we perceive reality. Yet there are some things we literally do not see, some questions we cannot ask. The job of research, Professor Smith concluded, is to punch holes in that screen.

Basic research into the nature and dynamics of "the third quarter of life" will have practical payoffs. As longevity has been extended during the course of this century, the adult prime also appears to have been lengthened. The vicissitudes of physical old age appear modifiable. That they can be delayed has been empirically demonstrated through clinical studies conducted in Sweden. Longstanding notions of the watershed points in adulthood and old age must be revised, therefore, for they no longer fit the reality of human experience (Svanborg, 1985). Adaptations in roles and norms over the life course perforce will transform basic societal rules.

An immediate task, therefore, is to gather quantitative and qualitative data on the physical, mental, psychological, occupational, and familial characteristics of men and women in the middle years of the life course, in order to reconstruct an historically sensitive model of adult development useful to policymakers, professionals, and scholars. Several tasks are obvious:

1. We need basic data. "The third quarter of life" is a catchy phrase, but it rests on little empirical or theoretical research. Should we really concentrate on the 25-year span between 50 and 75, or does it make more sense to encourage people over 40 (or men around one age and women at possibly another stage in their life course) to begin to take steps that will enable them to remain productive and active members of society? To address this cluster of questions will require analyzing a vast amount of survey and other data and then grappling with their meaning in both disciplinary and multidisciplinary manners.

2. We need to develop a stronger international perspective. Regrettably, the United States lags behind other advanced-industrial countries in attending seriously to the scope and components of a comprehensive aging policy. By thinking through our concerns with input from experts in Asia and Western Europe, we might be able to hasten our progress in this area.

3. We need to socialize and to train a more diverse group of American's present and future leaders to the problems and possibilities of an aging society, beginning with major curricula reforms among dental, educational, law, medical, public health, and social work faculties to introduce seminars and practice that take account of societal aging.

Admittedly, this net is cast widely. The three-point agenda clearly evolves from the radical hypothesis that societal aging will transform cultural values as well as socio-economic and political structures at a moment in history in which most Americans can expect to live longer. It should also be acknowledged that this thesis is not yet widely shared among other historians. The current "best seller" is *The Rise and Fall of Great Powers* (1987). The rise of the western world, according to Paul Kennedy, is due to economic and military breakthroughs; nations fall because the cost of sustaining military resources outstrips most available economic resources, thus making them unable to compete when new centers of production rise. Kennedy apparently discounts the significance of individual and societal aging: he underplays cultural matters (including the influence of values and attitudes on people's behavior) and demographic changes (such as the impact of plagues and declines in fertility rates). Hereafter, however, it will be reckless for researchers of the contemporary scene to be so cavalier. And therein lies the rub: we *know* we should take "age" seriously, but we really are not sure how to do it. To elaborate what I mean, I shall now turn to the second part of my essay. I hope to demonstrate that even in one of the nation's premier centers for research on aging, a certain agnosticism pervades intellectual discourse—for understandable reasons!

THE FUTURE OF GERONTOLOGY AMIDST DISCIPLINARY WATERSHEDS

Gerontology at The University of Michigan has been spearheaded for nearly half a century by a cadre of talented people whose vision transcended the classroom and their own particular research interests. Each of them—differences in scholarly careers and managerial styles notwithstanding—seized every promising opportunity to build bridges within and beyond the university community. Key moments in the development of academic gerontology at The University of Michigan reflect or presage shifting currents in the pursuit of knowledge and research dollars. They also correspond to new initiatives in the public-policy and social-service areas for applying research in addressing the problems of the elderly. Because these individuals were determined to create a center of excellence while laboring under difficult academic and organizational constraints, all sought to position the Institute at the cutting edge of change.

By doing a little bit of everything that was expected or that was in vogue, Michigan's gerontologists managed in the past to be all things to all constituencies. The present environment is not conducive to this strategy. But if we are to fulfill our mission in a different manner, particularly in light of the priorities of an aging society, we must confront issues that have always shadowed the emergence of gerontology as an academic specialty.

From the start, gerontology's intellectual turf was broadly defined. Old age, John Dewey (1939) declared, was a "*problem* and one of a scope having no precedent in human history...we need to know the ways in which social contexts react back into biological processes as well as to know the ways in which biological processes condition social life." Characterizing old age as a "problem" struck a responsive chord: by the late 1930s, most Americans believed that myriad physical woes and socio-economic vicissitudes made growing older a pitiable plight. The elderly's growing numbers and increasing vulnerability, moreover, posed a threat to the well-being of society at large (Haber, 1983; Achenbaum, 1983). But this was the heyday of intellectuals flocking to Washington and of college graduates assuming professional tasks in which they hoped to use their expertise in solving major challenges. Surely the opportunity to define and grapple with a problem bound to attract increasing attention nationwide would appeal to men and women eager to make their mark.

And yet, precisely because old age was a problem of unprecedented scope, scholars and academic entrepreneurs had difficulty fitting it into existing arrangements. The phenomenon and process of senescence clearly had biomedical, socio-economic, psychological, and practical dimensions. This meant, as Dewey suggested, that gerontologists would have to be concerned with the "big picture." University professors and scientists were not well-equipped, however, to tackle a novel and multifaceted problem like aging in a cross-disciplinary manner that presupposed collaboration with experts and practitioners outside of the university. For nearly half a century, the dominant trend within higher education had been toward narrower and narrower specialization (Veysey, 1965). Each discipline and professional school preferred to determine its own rules and set its own standards. Since aging is multifaceted, no single discipline perforce could preempt the fledgling field of gerontology.

Under the circumstances, the most sensible course of action was to foster the creation and diffusion of usable knowledge about aging. The immediate challenge was two-fold. On the one hand, the first generation of gerontologists had to persuade their colleagues that the intellectual and social problems associated with old age were so formidable as to justify concerted scholarly attention. On the other hand, those who wanted to advance the study of aging had to demonstrate that applying basic research would ameliorate the quality of later life. Without a reigning paradigm, the first generation of researchers adopted strategies that enabled them to capitalize on their previous scholarly endeavors and to tap resources available to them on the local scene. In this respect, the pioneers of gerontology, in retrospect, seem similar to those who advanced craniofacial biology as "normal science" (Carlson, 1985).

RESEARCH IN GERONTOLOGY: MICHIGAN'S INSTITUTE OF GERONTOLOGY

Over time, a gap between social science and biomedical research in gerontology evolved. The University of Michigan became a center of excellence in social gerontology, largely because two people—Clark Tibbitts and Wilma Donahue—succeeded in implementing an ambitious program of research, training, and service (Tibbitts, 1960). Nonetheless, it must be noted that gerontology still was a marginal intellectual activity here well into the 1960s. Marginality, for social gerontologists, was a double-edged sword. Because they did not have to compete for resources in the mainstream, a small group of talented, dedicated individuals could blaze frontiers of knowledge as they saw fit. Yet their valiant efforts did not automatically win them prestige or any comparative advantage on native soil: the real measure of their success would come when scholars across traditional disciplines began to engage in basic research on aging. Gerontology had to be accepted as a legitimate field of inquiry by the academy's gatekeepers.

Government legislated the aging enterprise before there was a critical mass of scholarship. Gerontology at Michigan entered its second stage in 1965, when John B. Martin, who headed the State Commission on Aging, recommended the establishment of an Institute of Gerontology jointly sponsored at The University of Michigan and Wayne State University. Dr. Donahue became the first director of the new Institute, which received an appropriation of $200,000 for its first year of operation The Institute was broadly charged with "developing new and improved programs (1) for helping older people in this state, (2) for training persons skilled in working with problems with the aged, (3) for research related to the needs of the aged, (4) and for conducting community services" (Eaton, 1981). A large training grant from the United States Administration on Aging in 1966-67 enabled the new Institute to establish a national reputation in the areas of curriculum development and text writing as it developed educational programs for social service and health care practitioners at the state level.

During Harold Johnson's tenure as the Ann Arbor branch's director in the 1970s, the Institute of Gerontology (IoG) greatly augmented state appropriations with "soft" money. It also reached out to encourage members of The University of Michigan's faculty to pursue research on aging under IoG auspices. Building on a network that existed in the Schools of Education, Public Health, and Social Work, teams were assembled to address topics ranging from minority aging, to legal issues affecting the aged (including elder abuse), to cross-national studies of the organization of health care services. The IoG received favorable publicity for projects that incorporated humanistic perspectives on aging, an area which was just beginning to attract scholarly attention nationwide.

By the beginning of the 1980s, the IoG was clearly perceived as one of few truly preeminent multidisciplinary centers in the nation that engaged in training, service, and research on aging. No overriding intellectual paradigm informed activities at the Institute, but at the time it really did not seem to matter. This was a period of growth and ferment. That new ideas were always circulating in the halls and programs were carried off with panache is a tribute to the ability of an energetic band of women and men to work well together in a fluid and high-pressured environment. They enjoyed attacking myths of aging through research; with almost evangelical fervor they were prepared to recruit and socialize people to work in the field. The Institute also benefited from the prestige and continuing activities of past and current directors and friends well placed at the state and federal levels.

Paradoxically, the Institute's most appealing strengths were also the source of two vulnerabilities in the eyes of hard-nosed researchers and professors in mainline disciplines at Michigan. First, no one could deny the importance of continuing education and outreach programs to benefit the elderly. It was these ventures, after all, that primarily interested state and federal funding agencies. Still, as economic cutbacks everywhere forced faculty committees and university administrators to review campus priorities mindful of fiscal exigencies, it was reasonable to ask whether the Institute would long continue to enjoy a comparative advantage in these areas over Michigan State University, Eastern Michigan University or other schools. Second, a "Directory of Aging Related Research" issued by the Institute in August 1982 listed 227 U-M researchers who were investigating aspects of aging. But, to put the matter bluntly, there were no outstanding researchers on the Institute's full-time staff in a university that operates on a "star" system.

It is too early to assess the impact of Richard Adelman's leadership on gerontology at Michigan, but it was clear upon his arrival that he intended to redirect priorities. Thus far Adelman has enunciated four major goals:

To put a primary emphasis on research. "Disciplinary rigor is an absolute requirement for high quality research and education, even in gerontology," Adelman declared (1983).

To insinuate the IoG program into the health arena. A central thrust has been to expand laboratory research in the biomedical sciences, to develop first-rate academic programs in geriatric health care, and to launch new initiatives in long-term care and health-services research.

To emphasize the research component of all educational endeavors, thus focusing on pre- and post-doctoral training.

To establish an Aging Society Policy Center. Issues such as the problems of older workers in an advanced-industrial economy, the needs of older women amid the feminization of poverty, the significance of race in the American version of the welfare state, and the organization and delivery of health care do not exist in a vacuum. Rather, these policy problems need to be investigated as they really exist, that is, in the context of "an aging society."

Adelman's vision has its exciting possibilities, particularly if multidisciplinary research efforts are indeed becoming a distinguishing characteristic of gerontology. But more systematic efforts will be needed to create a pliable vocabulary and a common frame of reference that will facilitate collaborative research. Effective communication across traditional disciplinary boundaries remains more of a goal than a reality. Gerontologists and the IoG must make explicit those elements of our personal methodologies that colleagues seem to share. "Vital paradigms are the property of communities of scientific practitioners who coalesce around them and are used both to generate and to solve puzzles," observed Busse and Maddox (1985). "Cumulatively, research concerning the shared paradigms generates a visible research tradition. Scientific revolutions, or more modestly, significant theoretical advances, occur when a community of scientists recognizes new puzzles it believes to be solvable and worth solving."

There are at least three such commonalities in work done by IoG faculty-researchers that might lead us to create a "vital paradigm":

1. Each is interested in the process of aging, not just the aged. Hitherto, there was an age-specific bias built into research at the Institute; scholars dealt with things old. Increasingly, however, IoG research scientists are looking at the nature and dynamics of bio-social processes at earlier stages of the life span because this facilitates their ability to pinpoint what is distinctive about the later stages of growth. Most gerontologists thus should acknowledge their affinity to developmentalists.

2. "Time" is an important independent variable in each of our research agendas. To what extent do things happen at the cellular, molecular, systemic, or societal level simply because the time clock keeps running, and processes set into motion evolve into different patterns? In what instances and under what conditions does the passage of time seem irrelevant—that is, when knowing how much time has elapsed from one

moment to another does not enhance one's likelihood of predicting that a certain event or process will occur. Does the rate of change matter?

3. Gerontological research is perforce comparative. Similarities and differences between "old" and "young" organisms matter greatly. So do continuities and changes over time. Indeed, whereas scholars in other disciplines can design research projects that eschew comparative elements, it is hard to think of an interesting topic in aging that does not presuppose some sort of control group or baseline by which one seeks to analyze results. At what level of abstraction should these comparisons be emphasized?

CONCLUSION: UNDERSTANDING THE AGING SOCIETY

A common set of research principles that define and operationalize "age" are a necessary resource for investigators in their individual and collective work. Research scientists might be able to develop a way to bridge the multiplicity of their research interests if they seek such common ground.

Deliberately fostering a community of discourse may enable gerontologists to grapple with issues that have bedeviled the development of this field of inquiry from the start: the tensions between basic and applied research; the points of divergence and convergence among biomedical, psycho-social, and humanistic perspectives on aging; and the proper balance between discipline-specific foci and multidisciplinary perspectives. If we can reach consensus on such thorny matters, then we will have done far more than our predecessors to define fundamental terms such as "age," "aging," and "aged."

All scientists and clinicians interested in aging critically need a developmentalist model that is at once sensitive to continuities and changes over time while being insistent on comparative analysis. That vantage point should serve us well as we seek to refine and redefine those intellectual skills that people require as they explore the frontiers of individual and societal aging in years to come. And, to bring this essay full circle, it is this intellectual challenge that makes "aging society" a fine intellectual template for this volume. More than ever before, we have a real interest in advancing our knowledge about basic facts of life. This is truly a brave new world, but one that is comprehensible only if we are willing to apply time-honored tools of intellectual reason and scientific inquiry.

REFERENCES

Achenbaum, W.A. *Old Age in the New Land.* Johns Hopkins University Press, Baltimore, 1978.

Achenbaum, W.A. *Shades of Gray.* Little, Brown and Co., Boston, 1983.

Achenbaum, W.A. Can gerontology be a science? J. Aging Studies *1:*3-18, 1987.

Adelman, R.C. A message from the Institute director. Institute of Gerontology, The University of Michigan, Ann Arbor, 1983.

Brown, C. and J.A. Pechman (Eds.) *Gender in the Workplace.* Brookings Institute, Washington, D.C., 1987.

Busse, E.W. and G.L. Maddox. *The Duke Longitudinal Studies of Normal Aging.* Springer Publishing, New York, 1985.

Calleo, D. *The Imperious Economy.* Harvard University Press, Cambridge, 1982.

Carlson, D.S. Craniofacial biology as normal science. In: *New Vistas in Orthodontics.* L.E. Johnston, Jr. (Ed.), Lea and Febiger, St. Louis, 1985.

Demos, J.P. *Past, Present, and Personal.* Oxford University Press, New York, 1986.

Dewey, J. Introduction. In: *Problems of Ageing.* E.V. Cowdy (Ed.), Williams and Wilkins, Baltimore, 1939.

Eaton (Miller), J. A synthesis of the history of the institute of gerontology. Institute of Gerontology, The University of Michigan, Ann Arbor, (unpub. mss.), 1981.

Friedan, B. *The Second Stage.* Summit Books, New York, 1981.

Haber, C. *Beyond Sixty-Five.* Cambridge University Press, New York, 1983.

Hagestad, G. Continuity and connectedness. In: *Grandparenthood.* V.L. Bergston and J.F. Robertson (Eds.), Sage Publications, Beverly Hills, 1985.

Haskell, T. (Ed.). *The Authority of Experts.* Indiana University Press, Bloomington, 1984.

Sorensen, A.B., R.E. Weinert, and L.E. Sherrod (Eds.). *Human Development and the Life Course.* Lawrence Erlbaun, Hillsdale, N.J., 1986.

Jones, L.Y. *Great Expectations.* Ballantine, New York, 1980.

Kennedy, P. *The Rise and Fall of The Great Powers.* Random House, New York, 1987.

Lasch, C. *Culture of Narcissism.* W. W. Norton, New York, 1979.

Longman, P. *Born to Pay.* Houghton Mifflin Company, Boston, 1987.

Maddox, G.L. and R.T. Campbell. Scope, concepts, and methods in the study of aging. In: *Handbook of Aging and The Social Sciences.* 2nd Ed., R.H. Binstock and E. Shanas (Eds.), Van Nostrand Reinhold, New York, 1985.

Neugarten, B.L. and D.A. Neugarten. Changing meanings of age in an aging society. In: *Our Aging Society.* A. Pifer and L. Bronte (Eds.), W.W. Norton, New York, 1986.

Pifer, A. The public policy response. In: *Our Aging Society.* A. Pifer and L. Bronte (Eds.), W.W. Norton, New York, 1986.

Riley, M.W. and J.W. Riley, Jr. Longevity and social structure. In: *Our Aging Society.* A. Pifer and L. Bronte (Eds.), W.W. Norton, New York, 1986.

Rossi, A.S. (Ed.). *Gender and the Life Course.* Aldine Publishing, Hawthorne, New York, 1985.

Starr, P. *The Social Transformation of American Medicine.* Basic Books, New York, 1982.

Svanborg, A. Biomedical and environmental influences on aging. In: *Productive Aging.* R.N. Burtler and H.P. Gleason (Eds.), Springer Publishing, New York, 1985.

Tibbitts, C. Origins, scope and fields of social gerontology. In: *Handbook of Social Gerontology.* C. Tibbitts (Ed.), University of Chicago Press, Chicago, 1960.

Torres-Gil, F. Hispanics in an aging society. In: *Our Aging Society.* A. Pifer and L. Bronte (Eds), W.W. Norton, New York, 1986.

U.S. Bureau of Census. *Demographic and Socioeconomic Aspects of Aging in the United States.* Series P-23, Government Printing Office, Washington, D.C., 1984.

Veroff, J., E. Douvan and R.A. Kulka. *The Inner American.* Basic Books, New York, 1981.

Veysey, L.R. *The Emergence of the American University.* University of Chicago Press, Chicago, 1965.

Wilson, W.J. *The Truly Disadvantaged.* University of Chicago Press, Chicago, 1987.

DENTAL PRACTICE IN THE AGING SOCIETY

Brian A. Burt

The aging of American society no longer makes news. The facts are well-known: the median age is now over 30 years of age for the first time, and the proportion of persons over the age of 65 will soon constitute over 20 percent of the U.S. population, with a considerably larger percentage of the population by the year 2010. These statements are neither speculative forecasts nor the results of some statistical exercise; the people concerned are already with us. What is still difficult for most of us, however, is to think through the implications of this demographic change for all of our societal institutions. As Dr. Achenbaum reminds us in this volume, "The inexorable aging of America's population will affect every institution in our society and the ways people live in the twenty-first century." Not only the way they live, it might be added, but also the way they think about themselves and the way they perceive and relate to the world around them.

Dental practice is just one of those institutions that will inevitably be affected, whether we prepare for it or not. In this paper I would like to present a brief assessment, from the viewpoint of an epidemiologist in oral disease, of how disease trends and social forces related to aging might combine to influence the practice of dentistry by the early years of the next century.

TRENDS IN ORAL DISEASE

There are essentially three current issues in oral health status, all somewhat interrelated, which together will strongly influence the conduct of dental practice in the years to come. The first is the decline in dental caries among children due to widespread use of fluorides over the last 20 or so years. Many teenagers and young adults today have never experienced "the drill" or a "shot in the mouth," and have probably never given a thought to possible loss of teeth. So long as fluoride use remains near its current levels, the incidence of caries is likely to remain low. A second oral disease issue today is the realization that generalized periodontitis, serious enough to threaten the dentition, is not as widespread as was once thought. The third issue is increasing tooth retention among older people, a trend which will become even more pronounced as the "caries-free" generation grows older, and which is worthy of some particular consideration.

Tooth Retention

Edentulism has been virtually synonymous with old age for so long in this country that it has shaped dental practice and attitudes towards older patients in a number of ways. Among the general public, loss of teeth was long considered a normal aspect of aging, something that went with wrinkles and sensory diminution. What is less well appreciated is that this attitude was shared by dentists as well, although for them it was wrapped up in the biological justification of "focal infection" (Burt, 1985). Patients came to their dentists expecting to have their remaining teeth out, and dentists, with the best of intentions, were usually prepared to oblige. In the earlier years of this century, when the scientific basis for dental practice was poor, the technology available to dentists primitive, and dentistry was struggling toward recognition as a profession, it was hardly surprising that the vast majority of older people became totally edentulous. The lifetime dental pathway for most people went from tooth decay in childhood, with some tooth loss and some fillings, through additional toothaches and gum disease in adulthood, until the time was reached when "having them all out" was seen as the sensible thing to do.

Attitudinal Changes

But most older people now are maintaining their dentitions and will continue to do so to an increasing degree; the proportion of people who have lost all their teeth will continue to decline slowly until it reaches an irreducible low point around the year 2020 (Weintraub and Burt, 1985). The earlier pathway toward tooth loss just described is not seen as the norm today, so what has changed? The changes most obvious to those in the dental profession are the expansion of the scientific basis for dental practice and technological advances. Although there is no question that developments in these areas have been profound, social changes, and the shifts in attitudes that followed them, have had effects that are just as extensive.

THE "NEW ELDERLY"

Perhaps the greatest social change is the emergence of the group that has been called the "new elderly," meaning those individuals 65 years of age or older who are active, healthy, and most of all dentate (Ettinger and Beck, 1982). Throughout the period during which good national statistics on oral health status have been kept, the elderly in the United States were those whose life experiences were shaped by the depression of the 1930s, when expectations were naturally modest. That period was followed by World War II, which did little to expand these expectations; indeed many young men became edentulous in the armed forces at that time as a "dental expediency." Attitudes shaped during these traumatic years did not easily change, even when times got better. Many who had not already lost all their teeth accepted their eventual edentulous state with passive resignation; it was what they expected.

But those turning 65 today are essentially a post-war generation. Their formative times were the post-war "boom" years, when national expectations were almost boundless and the affluent era brought dental care increasingly within the reach of many who would not have previously considered it an option. Utilization of dental care was increasing during the 1950s and 1960s, prior to the era of widespread dental insurance. This was also the time when systematic and well-funded dental research began in earnest, and technological advances in equipment and materials jumped ahead. The "focal infection" theory passed into history, and the modern age of tooth retention began around that time.

FUTURE IMPACT ON DENTAL PRACTICE

It is not difficult to think of many areas in society which will be profoundly affected by the aging population. One obvious area is Social Security. When the first Social Security Act was passed during the depression emergency in 1935, the average life expectancy was 68 years of age and the population structure was slanted toward younger people. Planners of the system, therefore, established it to fit the needs of the time. Today's situation, with life expectancy some 10 years longer and with an inverted population structure, is radically different. This is the principal reason why the Social Security system, as originally devised, will come under increasing strain as time goes by.

But to look ahead to dental practice by the early years of the next century, the biggest influence will probably come from that group known as the "baby-boomers," the bulge in the population curve from the high-fertility post-war period between 1947 and 1963. As it moves through its lifespan, that group has forced a number of social adjustments, beginning with pressure on schools, then on colleges, the job market, and housing. The social adaptation required when this group reaches elderly status is likely to be even greater. The first wave of the "baby-boomers" is now in its 40s, and so by early next century will be approaching its mid-60s. There are probably a number of things we can expect from this group as it begins to swell the ranks of the elderly at that time.

While the "yuppie" image of the acquisitive young adult may well be a stereotype, it is true that this particular generation has grown up in a period of more widespread affluence and higher expectations than have previously been known in human history. Whole industries have sprung up catering to the wants of this generation. Just as the attitudes of the depression/World War II group did not easily change as its members grew older, it is reasonable to expect that the attitudes of the baby-boomers will not change much either. At the risk of stereotyping, it can be said that, perhaps more than any other generation, this group has been preoccupied with appearance and self-image; perhaps that, too, is unlikely to change. When added to the changing trends in oral diseases discussed earlier, the picture of the elderly baby-boomers in the next century emerges as one of a generation whose dental demands will be little different from those of young adults today. It can also be expected that this group will be enjoying longer life expectancy, which might average over 80 years by the next century.

These evolutionary changes in dental attitudes will be part of what is likely to be the most radical attitudinal shift of all, which is the notion that 65 or 70 years of age is no longer old. While there are current examples of older persons whose behavior diverges from that associated with traditional elderly roles (through, for example, continuing their education, pursuing athletic endeavors, or having non-traditional tastes in music), this trend is likely to be much more commonplace by the next century. The upper boundary of "middle age" will be extended further than it is now, and the very concept of aging will be redefined.

Dental practice since the 1950s has focused on restorative care in children, a focus which is now fading with the caries decline in children. Dental care will increasingly become a process spread more evenly through life than it has been. Just as many "family" practices were geared mainly toward children's dentistry, the demographic inversions of our time will require such practices to give much more attention to older persons. This trend is distinct from the welcome attention now being given to "geriatric dentistry," with its emphasis on treatment of institutionalized individuals, for it will have as its focus a large number of healthy, active, and reasonably affluent patients between 60 and 80 years of age.

The best way to anticipate the dental demands of this sizable group, therefore, is to consider the dental demands of young adults today. Restorations (first-time or replacements), crowns and bridges, periodontal prophylaxes, and orthodontic care are the areas of greatest demand in this group, and it is likely that these will be the areas for which future demand for dental care will come from older people. Orthodontic care for this group, therefore, may be as common then as it is today for young adults.

These major shifts in demography and disease distribution are already having an impact on dental practice, and they will continue to do so. The future for dental practice, however, conducted in a population in which levels of oral health will be higher even than today's, remains bright.

REFERENCES

Burt, B.A. The oral health of older Americans. Am. J. Public Health (editorial). *75:*1133-1134, 1985.

Ettinger, R.L. and J.D. Beck. The new elderly: What can the dental profession expect? Special Care Dent. *2:*62-69, 1982.

Weintraub, J.A. and B.A. Burt. Tooth loss in the United States. J. Dent. Educ. *49:*368-376, 1985.

MYTHS AND REALITIES OF BIOLOGICAL AGING

Richard C. Adelman

The outer limits of longevity appear to be genetically determined. However, the proportion of a population that survives to approach its maximal life span is highly dependent on environmental factors. Numerous functional capabilities change during aging; some for the better and some for the worse. However, at least many deficits in performance represent artifacts of disease and lifestyle. What is the potential for human performance and survival if it becomes possible to maintain good health and the integrity of functional capability throughout the life span? Highlights of successes and stumbling blocks which thus far characterize research on the biology of aging are the subject of the article.

DETERMINANTS OF THE LIFESPAN

Longevity

Most of what was known about human longevity until the early 1960s can be gleaned from reading the survival statistics of various populations (Comfort, 1956). For example, in British India during the 1920s, the average individual had a life expectancy of approximately 25 to 30 years, whereas the oldest individual lived approximately 100 years. In New Zealand during the mid 1930s, the average individual had a life expectancy of approximately 75 to 80 years, whereas the oldest individual also lived approximately 100 years; these are remarkably similar to more current statistics for the U.S.A. (Brody and Brock, 1985).

A reasonable interpretation of these kinds of data is that there probably are environmental and genetic determinants of human longevity. As the environment improves, the average individual is characterized by a greater life expectancy. Typical environmental improvements might include better medical care, high technology, sanitation, nutritional behavior, social counseling, and so forth. At the same time, throughout recorded human history, apparent maximal lifespan has remained approximately the same: somewhat in excess of 100 years. What has changed is the percentage of the human population that approaches the apparent maximal lifespan. This observation, as well as many other data such as the species-specific nature of apparent maximal lifespan, lends support to the notion that there probably also is a genetic component to longevity.

The implications of these observations for the health care establishment, recently reviewed (Brody and Brock, 1985), are both intriguing and controversial, although detailed discussion of this subject is beyond the scope of this article. Some interpret the changing nature of human life expectancy as support for the notion that the optimal medical accomplishment is survival in good health until the clock strikes twelve on the final day of the final year of the genetically endowed lifespan. Perhaps the practice of preventive medicine will compress morbidity to only the most trivial portion of the very end of maximal lifespan. On the other hand, there are considerable data which support the likelihood that society can look forward to increasing numbers of very old, chronically ill people. For example, mortality rates for both men and women older than 75 years are declining precipitously.

The complexities of human longevity only are beginning to become apparent. Consider the following select examples.

1. In several geographic regions of the world, there are isolated mountainous areas containing people who claim to live as long as 130-150 years of age (Comfort, 1979). It has become increasingly evident that inaccurate birth records, as well as nationalistic chauvinism, contribute significantly to these inappropriate claims.

2. Premature aging is attributed to those unfortunate children who appear perfectly normal as newborn infants, but who acquire many physical symptoms of old age and die during their early teens of a complicated set of illnesses lumped under the term progeria (Comfort, 1979). However, there are symptoms of progeria that present quite differently than those of old age.

3. The increased number of women who are dying of lung cancer attributable to cigarette smoking may begin to erode the well-established longer life expectancy of women relative to men (Glynn and Cullen, 1985; Miller and Gerstein, 1983; Surgeon General's Report, 1980).

4. Old men who are married to younger women live longer than old men who are married to older women (Foster *et al.,* 1984).

Biological Studies of Longevity

Why does one species of animal or plant live longer than another? Putting this question in slightly different terms, how does a researcher whose productive laboratory lifespan is 25 years (minus administrative inclinations) design experiments that are to contribute to the body of information on the basis of the human lifespan that exceeds 100 years?

One experimental approach to identifying factors that affect the length of the lifespan was provided by the prominent cell biologist, Leonard Hayflick, during the early 1960s (Hayflick and Moorhead, 1961). He and his colleagues observed that normal human cells grown in culture survive for a specific period of time. When normal, embryonic lung tissue is exposed to a carefully defined environment *in vitro*, cells begin to grow until a single monolayer of cells covers the surface of the piece of laboratory glassware in which the tissue was placed. When the monolayer of cells is scraped off the surface of the glassware, divided into two equal portions, and placed into two new pieces of laboratory glassware of the same size and shape, cell division resumes until two monolayers are formed, and cell division ceases once again. In other words, these manipulations cause the cell population to double. The original important observation by Hayflick in these experiments, which has been confirmed by numerous other researchers, is that the cell population doubles only 50 times, plus or minus biological variation, and then the cells die.

Based on these observations, it was suggested that the phenomenon of finite lifespan is expressed at the level of isolated normal cells grown in culture. Support for this concept subsequently was provided by the additional observations that cells isolated from older individuals exhibit less proliferative capacity than do cells isolated from younger individuals (Martin *et al.,* 1970) and that cells isolated from longer-lived species exhibit a greater proliferative capacity than do cells isolated from shorter-lived species (Rohme, 1981). Currently, numerous laboratories are utilizing this cellular model system in efforts to isolate and to characterize senescence-specific genes.

BIOLOGICAL PROCESSES OF AGING

Two general kinds of issues characterize research in this area. One concerns afflictions of elderly individuals. The other addresses the origin and sequence of developmental events which ultimately are expressed as the progressively changing ability to adapt to environmental challenges throughout the lifespan.

Until very recently, most physiological assessments painted an entirely depressing picture of functional decline in elderly people. Such a view is based on enormous quantities of data that indicate that physiological capabilities are progressively lost during aging. Select examples of such data, collected primarily by Nathan Shock and colleagues, include rate of blood flow through the kidney, speed of nerve impulses, and so forth (Shock, 1960). In virtually every system studied, mean values decline with increasing human age beyond 30 years.

Recently, the difficulty of interpretation of these data has become more fully appreciated. For example, there was enormous variation about the mean values. In other words, there always were individuals among the oldest age groups who performed as well as those from the youngest age groups. Furthermore, virtually all of the earlier assessments were derived from cross-sectional studies, in which the role of cohort effects could not be examined.

It is becoming increasingly evident that many of the impaired physiological capabilities associated with old age in humans probably are not consequences of intrinsic biological processes of aging. Instead, they probably reflect the effects of disease, inappropriate diet and levels of exercise, and uninformed social policy. Each of the following three examples reinforce this key message.

Sexual Activity and Aging. Perhaps the single most notable example is the issue of sexual activity, which until very recently was generally depicted in virtually all medical and physiological textbooks as a functional capability that declines during aging. The experimental basis of such dogma had been the progressively diminished level of circulating testosterone in aging men. However, careful examination of the primary research literature indicates that, until fairly recently, studies were based on measurements obtained from institutionalized men who were sick and/or segregated from women. More recent investigations (Warner *et al.,* 1985), based on measurements from healthy elderly men who either are community-dwelling or institutionalized, but socialized with women, reveal that both testosterone levels and sexual activity can remain undiminished until as late as 60 to 80 years of age. Therefore, the well-intentioned, frugal, or puritanistic policy decision of many years ago not to house men and women in the same room within long-term care institutions actually provoked a biological change which routinely and inappropriately was accepted as a biomarker of aging.

Glucose Intolerance and Aging. A second example of questionable physiological decline during aging is glucose intolerance, which, until very recently was also depicted in virtually all medical and physiological textbooks as a necessary feature of aging. It is now generally recognized that glucose intolerance during aging is greatly accentuated by diabetes and obesity, and that it can be minimized when healthy elderly people are subjected to the appropriate regimen of diet and exercise (Chen *et al.,* 1987; Reaven and Reaven, 1980).

Cardiac Performance and Aging. Yet another example of dogma associated with the aging process is that of cardiac performance. Virtually all medical and physiological textbooks, until very recently, depicted cardiac performance as progressively and inevitably diminished during aging. Recent improvements in the ability to diagnose cardiac disease, however, revealed that healthy elderly people are not characterized by declining cardiac performance (Lakatta, 1985).

Adaptation and the Aging Process

One general feature that does seem to characterize all aging individuals is a progressively modified ability to adapt to changes in the surrounding environment. For example, the effectiveness of intragastrically administered glucose in enhancing the synthesis of the liver enzyme glucokinase progressively diminishes with aging in rats for which genetics and environment are rigorously controlled (Adelman, 1970). In other words, the more familiar sluggish response by elderly pedestrians who attempt to avoid oncoming cars is also expressed at the molecular level by the sluggish biosynthesis of a specific gene product (glucokinase) when a particular cell population (the hepatocyte) of the intact organism (rat) is challenged by ingestion of a nutrient (glucose). In this particular example, the altered regulation of hepatic enzyme synthesis during aging apparently reflects an imbalance of the pancreatic hormones, insulin, glucagon and somatostatin (Adelman and Freeman, 1972; Adelman, 1975; Sartin *et al.,* 1980; Chaudhuri *et al.,* 1983). The chronological origin of these endocrine changes apparently is near birth (Adelman, 1970). Therefore, an important goal of this research is identification of the events that occur at early ages that program progressive change in physiological capability throughout the remainder of the lifespan. It should be recognized that this approach to gerontological research represents the efforts to understand the adaptive regulation of only one of dozens of such known enzyme changes during aging, and that it is only one example of a number of different experimental approaches to the understanding of gerontological change.

LIKELIHOOD OF INTERVENTION IN THE AGING PROCESS

Successful intervention in aging was achieved in rats more than 50 years ago when it was demonstrated that moderate restriction of the dietary intake of *ad libitum* fed rats results in an apparent doubling of the maximal lifespan (McCay *et al.,* 1935). More recently it was demonstrated that not only the quantity but also the quality of life are improved when rats are subjected to moderate diet restriction (Masoro, 1985). Many of the diseases and functional changes that characterize old *ad libitum* fed rats also are expressed in diet-restricted animals, but not until much later ages.

Clinical Implications

The clinical implications of these data are both intriguing and controversial. Naturally, medical ethics prevent us from similarly restricting the diets of people. However, it seems reasonable to suggest that if a regimen of diet and exercise has the potential to improve the quality and quantity of human life, then this result would have been demonstrated by now, at least in certain segments of the American population. Such a result has not yet been produced, although there are numerous advocates of adopting diet and exercise regimens. Perhaps relevant data are represented by individuals who are at great risk of death by cardiovascular failure, for whom the appropriate regimen of diet and exercise produces significant improvements in the quantity and quality of life expectancy (Weber *et al.,* 1983). This is by no means the same as extending the duration of the viable lifespan of rats by diet restriction. However, it does seem to indicate that the quality and quantity of human life may be susceptible to nutritional manipulation.

On the other hand, there also are data suggesting that moderate obesity is a positive determinant of longevity. For example, recent longitudinal studies indicate that moderately obese men who do not die of heart attacks during their early 50s, although at greater risk of diabetes, hypertension and so forth, live longer than leaner counterparts (Andres *et al.,* 1985). What better substantiation of this finding can one request than the recent upward revision of ideal body weights by the Metropolitan Life Insurance Company (Harrison, 1985)?

SOCIETAL IMPACT OF RESEARCH ON AGING

What is the potential societal impact of successful biomedical research in gerontology? This topic requires examination in far greater depth than is possible in this article. Perhaps the most effective means to broach the subject is to imagine the discovery of an elixir which can painlessly and quickly convert old rats into young rats. Imagine further the consternation expressed by that first person who self-administers the elixir, only to discover that he or she, too, is painlessly and quickly converted into a young rat.

This approach to a discussion of the societal impact of biomedical research in gerontology is an historically successful one for several reasons. (1) It generally is appreciated as humor. (2) It allows one to moralize, at least to the extent that it is important to advocate cautious interpretation of the results of gerontological experiments. (3) It encourages, in a gerontological context, resurrection of the suggestion that some research is perhaps best left undone, and that there may be more potential danger than benefit to humanity as a consequence of the accumulation of certain kinds of knowledge (Sinsheimer, 1978).

There are many who believe that our society does not yet know how to house, feed, clothe and otherwise care for our most frail elderly citizens. Given this state of affairs, how shall society deal with an even greater proportion of such individuals in the event that biomedical research extends the human lifespan without substantial improvement in the quality of life? An equally important view concerns the growing number of productive, healthy elderly people within developed and developing countries of the world. In this case, the need for change is just as evident, although substantively different, pointing instead to intergenerational problems at the workplace and home, the cost of social and health care, targets for the educational and advertising enterprises, and so forth.

While it is responsible to raise questions about the values that are embodied in various aspects of gerontological research, excessive caution could tend to inhibit the search for new knowledge and impede progress in developing the pathway to enlightenment. Communication that reaches across the disciplines and professions, as well as to the lay public, is absolutely necessary in the field of gerontology, which touches virtually every aspect of life. It is in this light that one should consider research on the biology of aging.

REFERENCES

Adelman, R.C. An age-dependent modification of enzyme regulation. J. Biol. Chem. *245:*1032-1035, 1970.

Adelman, R.C. and C. Freeman. Age-dependent regulation of glucokinase and tyrosine aminotransferase activities of rat liver *in vivo* by adrenal, pancreatic and pituitary hormones. Endocrinol. *90:*1551-1560, 1972.

Adelman, R.C. Impaired hormonal regulation of enzyme activity during aging. In: *Biology of Aging and Development.* G.J. Thorbecke (Ed.), Plenum Publishing Corporation, New York, 1975.

Andres, R., D. Elahi and J. Tobin. Impact of age on weight goals. Ann. Int. Med. *103(6):*1030-1033, 1985.

Brody, J.A. and D.B. Brock. Epidemiologic and statistical characteristics of the United States elderly population. In: *Handbook of Biology.* C.E. Finch and E.L. Schneider (Eds.), Van Nostrand Reinhold Co., New York, 1985.

Chen, M., J.B. Halter and D. Porte, Jr. The role of dietary carbohydrate in the decreased glucose tolerance of the elderly. J. Am. Geriatr. Soc. *35:*417-424, 1987.

Comfort, A. *The Biology of Senescence.* Holt, Rinehart and Winston, Inc., New York, 1956.

Comfort, A. *The Biology of Senescence.* 3rd Edition, Elsevier North Holland, Inc., New York, 1979.

Chaudhuri, M., J.L. Sartin and R.C. Adelman. A role for somatostatin in the impaired insulin secretory response to glucose by islets from aging rats. J. Gerontol. *38:*431-435, 1983.

Foster, D., L. Klinger-Vartabedian and L. Wispe. Male longevity and age differences between spouses. J. Gerontol. *39(1):*117-120, 1984.

Glynn, T.J. and J.W. Cullen. Smoking and women's health. In: *Women's Health, Report of the Public Health Service Task Force on Women's Health Issues.* Volume II. U.S. Dept. of Health and Human Services, May, 1985.

Harrison, G. Height-weight tables in health implications of obesity. Ann. Int. Med. *103(6):*989-994, 1985.

Hayflick, L. and P.S. Moorhead. The serial cultivation of human diploid cell strains. Exp. Cell. Res. *25:*585-621, 1961.

Lakatta, E.G. Heart and circulation. In: *Handbook of Biology of Aging.* C.B. Finch and E.L. Schneider (Eds.), Van Nostrand Reinhold Co., New York, 1985.

Martin, G.M., C.A. Sprague and C.J. Epstein. Replicative lifespan of cultivated human cells: Effects of donor's age, tissue and genotype. Lab. Invest. *23:*86-92, 1970.

Masoro, E.J. Metabolism. In: *Handbook of Biology of Aging.* C.E. Finch and E.L. Schneider (Eds.), Van Nostrand Reinhold Co., New York, 1985.

McCay, C.M., M.F. Crowell and L.A. Maynard. The effect of retarded growth upon the length of lifespan and upon the ultimate body size. J. Nutrition *10:*63-79, 1935.

Miller, G.H. and D.R. Gerstein. The life expectancy of nonsmoking men and women. Publ. Health Rep. *98:*343, 1983.

Reaven, E.P. and G.P. Reaven. Structure and function changes in the endocrine pancreas of aging rats with reference to the modulating effects of exercise and caloric restriction. J. Clin. Invest. *68:*75-84, 1981.

Rohme, D. Evidence for a relationship between longevity of animal species and lifespan of normal fibroblasts *in vitro* and erythrocytes *in vivo.* Proc. Natl. Acad. Sci. *78:*5009-5013, 1981.

Sartin, J., M. Chaudhuri, M. Obenrader and R.C. Adelman. The role of hormones in changing adaptive mechanisms during aging. Fed. Proc. *39:*3163-3167, 1980.

Shock, N.W. *Biology of Aging.* American Institute of Biological Sciences. Washington, D.C., 1960.

Sinsheimer, R. The presumptions of science. Daedalus *107:*23-35, 1978.

Surgeon General's Report. *The Health Consequences of Smoking for Women.* U.S. Dept. of Health and Human Services, 1980.

Warner, M., L. Dufau and R.J. Santen. Effects of aging and illness on the pituitary testicular axis in men: Qualitative as well as quantitative changes in luteinizing hormone. J. Clin. Endocrin. Metab. *60(2):*263-268, 1985.

Weber, F., R.J. Barnard and D. Roy. Effects of a high-complex-carbohydrate, low-fat diet and daily exercise on individuals 70 years of age and older. J. Gerontol. *38(2):*155-161, 1983.

DIRECTIONS OF AGING

Stanley M. Garn

The Model T Ford, with its planetary transmission, provided Americans of an earlier era with cheap transportation. The Model T also provided biologists with a simplistic model of aging. Since Model T's ran fine until some part wore out, it was natural to imagine that human aging was also due to the wearing out of parts! This quasi-mechanical explanation for aging is about as antique now as the "Flivver" itself, though not totally inapplicable to the human dentition.

Another approach to aging, less mechanistic and more biological, involves the life-cycle approach, measuring and recording dimensional and functional changes over the life span. Through this approach a great deal of descriptive information has been accumulated that relates not just to obvious decreases in size and function, but also to increases that are pathological in nature, and to some lifelong increases that may be normal, benign and even advantageous.

AGE-ASSOCIATED INCREASES

Among Americans and other westernized peoples, blood lipids increase with age, consistently and inexorably, so that septuagenarians are—as a group—hyperlipidemic. Serum cholesterol averages well over 200 mg/dl, a population value that we view with alarm. The triglycerides also increase with age, to approximately 200 mg/dl. This level is effectively close to hypertriglyceridemia, again far in excess of a "healthy" level, by any risk appraisal (Table 1).

As age increases in this group, both systolic and diastolic blood pressures rise, to the point where some 30 percent of septuagenarians are at least borderline hypertensive. Perhaps half of these individuals are prescribed anti-hypertensives or low-sodium diets or both; we have turned to the drug industry to control excessive lipid levels and increased blood pressure levels, in order to minimize the risk of cardiovascular demise.

Yet the rise in serum cholesterol, in the triglycerides, and in systolic and diastolic blood pressure is not necessarily the human condition. In

Table 1. Changes in weight, skinfolds, lipids, and blood pressure from 10 years of age to 75 years of age.

	Age, in years			
	10-14	15-19	20-49	50-75
	Males			
Number	196	337	1,443	603
Weight (kg)	47.08	69.92	79.95	78.50
Summed skinfold (mm)	49.81	57.20	84.45	84.42
Serum cholesterol (mg/dl)	163.48	161.02	198.27	210.85
Serum triglycerides (mg/dl)	100.48	125.77	194.27	200.09
Diastolic blood pressure (mm/Hg)	64.85	67.18	76.88	80.90
	Females			
Number	199	329	1,656	652
Weight (kg)	47.00	58.50	64.79	68.33
Summed skinfold (mm)	69.14	74.66	99.77	122.51
Serum cholesterol (mg/dl)	165.22	166.67	195.16	224.22
Serum triglycerides (mg/dl)	103.90	88.71	126.76	170.39
Diastolic blood pressure (mm/Hg)	65.06	68.07	74.23	79.48

Source: Tecumseh Community Health Survey, Examination Round 3. See also Garn *et al.,* 1988

certain populations, serum cholesterol stays under 100 mg/dl, triglycerides are comparably low, and blood pressure does not increase from age 20 to age 70. There are also populations in which fatness does not increase either, and in which septuagenarians are actually leaner than 20-year-olds. Moreover, some individuals do not increase in lipid or triglyceride or blood pressure values, to their cardiovascular fortune. What we know about "aging" from National Probability Surveys and in the U.S. or the U.K. may merely describe an increasing prevalence of pathology in high-risk modern populations.

THE DECREASES THAT GO WITH AGE

To be sure, there are many parameters that decrease with age. We all shrink in stature, from the 5th decade onward. In a study based on data collected in Tecumseh, Michigan, stature loss is half an inch from age

Table 2. Evidence for continuing bone expansion throughout life.

Hrdlička, 1936, 1938	Observed increase in hat size and inferred head size increase especially in "brainworkers"
Moore, 1955	Cross-sectional indications of continuing increase in cranial vault thickness
Smith and Walker, 1964	Cross-sectional radiographic evidence for femoral expansion in women
Epker, Kelin and Frost, 1965	Increase in rib cross-sectional area
Garn, Garn *et al.,* 1967, 1968, 1981	Continuing bone expansion in the metacarpals and other bones
Trotter and Peterson, 1968	Confirmation of continuing femoral expansion using skeletalized material
Israel, 1968, 1970, 1973, 1977, 1978	Continuing expansion of the vertebrae, the mandible and the cranial skeleton
Behrents, 1985, 1988	Using semi-longitudinal skull radiographs of 22,000 participants in the Bolton-Broadbent studies, extended our knowledge of lifelong bone expansion

50 to age 60 (Garn *et al.,* 1988). We all lose bone, from age 40 on, more rapidly if we are female and less rapidly if we are male (Garn, 1970). In consequence, we are at increasing risk of bone fracture and vertebral collapse. As the years go by, there are decreases in muscle mass, hemoglobin levels, and daily caloric requirements. No population has yet been found in which these decreases do not occur. Even the fossil hominids lost bone during their lifetimes, as did our subfossil ancestors, so bone loss is not a recent phenomenon of sedentary living or "modernization" (Garn, 1970).

CONTINUING BONE EXPANSION THROUGHOUT LIFE

It comes as a surprise to discover that even as we lose bone we also gain bone through continuing bone expansion. Hrdlička began to suspect this when his hat got too tight, but by that time he was a member of the National Academy of Sciences (Hrdlička, 1936, 1938). Moore nearly realized this in his important book *Hyperostosis Cranii* (1953). The orthopedist Harold Frost discovered continuing expansion of the femur, as did the endocrinologist Richmond Smith, Jr. (Table 2). They both attributed femoral expansion to the stimulus of weight-bearing on the principal weight-bearing long bones. We found bone expansion in the metacarpals, not weight-bearing bones in most of us (Garn *et al.,* 1967, 1968). Israel (1968) discovered it in the bones of the head (rarely weight bearing, except in Yoga practitioners). Behrents reports on the continuing expansion of the bones of the head and face in his paper in this volume. This is a new and important model of aging, contradicting the old notion that changes associated with aging inevitably involve decreases.

The reasons for continuing bone expansion at the outer surfaces of bones synchronic with bone loss at their inner surfaces are not known. It does occur in acromegaly, suggesting a role of human growth hormone (HGH) or somatomedin. It is mimicked in Paget's disease, though localized in the cranium and the middle digits in that disease. Continuing bone expansion is of paramount interest to orthodontists, who have long been habituated to teen-age dimensional norms, but who are now treating increasing numbers of adult and older adult patients.

SEX DIFFERENCES IN THE ONSET OF AGING

There are still other mysteries, surprises, and contradictions to be found in reviewing life-cycle dimensional and functional findings. One surprise is that the onset of "aging," traditionally identified as the beginning of the types of decrease mentioned above, is generally later in women than in men. Men experience decreases in hemoglobin and hematocrit levels rather early, by age 30 in some studies and by age 40 in others. In women, these levels continue to increase long after the age of 40. Hematologically speaking, women get better and better. Women also increase in fatness longer than men do, in the U.S.A. and comparable westernized countries. They continue to increase in lipid levels and in triglycerides longer than men do, for reasons that are not clear.

Logically, we would indeed expect an *earlier* onset of aging in females, who are developmentally advanced over males in nearly every measured phenomenon, beginning early in embryonic life. The female is advanced in odontogenesis, in tooth formation, in tooth eruption, and in attainment of the occlusal level. The female is systematically advanced over the male in ossification timing (by years, for some ossification centers), and attains reproductive maturity some 10% earlier than the male. That females attain emotional maturity earlier than males is also a common observation. Yet, despite developmental advancement from the first month of gestation through the age of legal adulthood, women experience physical manifestations of age later, not earlier, than men. And though women lose more bone than men do, both absolutely (measured in grams of bone) and relatively (expressed as a percentage), they are not earlier in the onset of adult bone loss.

Women also have an advantage over men in the duration of bone expansion, which continues from the end of the second decade through the tenth. Their tubular bones expand twice as much (9% vs. 4%) or twice as fast (1% vs. 0.5% per decade) as those of men. This may be a real advantage during the sixth decade, when continuing subperiosteal apposition may outpace endosteal surface resorption, leading to bones that are (transiently) bigger and stronger, though more hollow. Though diminished bone density (i.e., the amount of bone tissue in the anatomical bone) may be a disadvantage with respect to bending stress, continuing bone enlargement may convey a needed advantage in the presence of compressive forces.

IS AGING THE SAME AROUND THE WORLD?

It is very clear from the data of the Ten-State Nutrition Survey, NHANES-I and NHANES-II and the Tecumseh Community Health Survey that the course of aging and the onset of many age-associated declines differ between the sexes. Findings from these different studies, involving more than 60,000 participants, are consistent with life tables and population projections showing a longer life expectancy for the female. The cross-sectional data derived from the living and mortality experience are also consistent with life tables for many domestic animals. One might generalize and say that the female is programmed to live longer and that mortality experience simply reflects that fact. Just look at the sex ratio in any home for the aged, or among nonagenarians, or for those who pass the century mark. (Note the way insurance companies calculate two-person survivorship benefits from annuities when the spouses are of equal age!)

However, all of these cited data are for North Americans and they may not truly reflect the human condition. Though female longevity exceeds that of males now, by some 7 years—and this sex difference is increasing—it was not the case in the U.S.A. a century ago, and it is not the case in some third-world populations now.

Women have moved into the work place in growing numbers, exposing themselves to industrial chemicals and other occupational stresses. Some causes of death such as lung cancer are rising as the women who began to smoke during World War II reach the critical age. It may be that we will soon have to reconsider our notions about female longevity in general. It may also be that, despite occupational hazards, greater female longevity will continue and that we will have to uncover both the chromosomal and the hormonal factors involved.

AN EPISTLE TO ORTHODONTISTS

For this audience, in particular, I should not ignore the technical and operational challenges that an increasing cohort of the elderly necessarily provides. In addition to the challenge presented by the biology of "aging" and our personal desires to extend our life spans, we are faced with more and more older people with reasonably intact dentitions. They do not prefer prostheses, they do want to look good, and they are cognizant of cosmetic orthodontics. Though some have lost supporting bone and their tooth roots are fenestrating, many others have much supporting bone remaining. Moreover, as their jaws continue to grow, they need help in preserving occlusal relationships. This creates new needs and new opportunities. What are the normal dentofacial relationships for septuagenarians and octogenarians? How much do they differ from the teen-age norms long encapsulated in the literature? Do we now need to develop occlusal and dentofacial standards for those ages once considered beyond attainment for the majority of humans?

ACKNOWLEDGMENTS

This study was supported in part by a grant from the Weight Watchers Research Foundation. I wish to thank Cynthia Housh for her assistance in manuscript completion.

REFERENCES

Behrents, R.G. *An Atlas of Growth in the Aging Craniofacial Skeleton.* Monograph 18, Craniofacial Growth Series, Center for Human Growth and Development, University of Michigan, Ann Arbor, 1985.

Behrents, R.G. The consequences of adult craniofacial growth. In: *Orthodontics in an Aging Society.* Monograph 22, Craniofacial Growth Series, Center for Human Growth and Development, University of Michigan, Ann Arbor, 1989.

Cowdry, E.V. *Aging Better.* Charles C Thomas, Springfield, 1972.

Epker, B.N., M. Kelin and H.M. Frost. Magnitude and location of cortical bone loss in the human rib with aging. Clin. Orthop. *41:*198-203, 1965.

Garn, S.M., C.G. Rohmann, B. Wagner and W. Ascoli. Continuing bone growth throughout life: A general phenomenon. Am. J. Phys. Anthrop. *26:*313-318, 1967.

Garn, S.M., B. Wagner, C.G. Rohmann and W. Ascoli. Further evidence for continuing bone expansion. Am. J. Phys. Anthrop. *28:*219-222, 1968.

Garn, S.M. The earlier gain and later loss of cortical bone. Charles C Thomas, Springfield, 1970.

Garn, S.M. Contributions of the radiographic image to our knowledge of human growth. Am. J. Roentgen. *137:*231-239, 1981.

Garn, S.M., T.V. Sullivan, and V.M. Hawthorne. Age changes in hard and soft tissues and lipids. N.Y. Med. Quarterly *8:*40-46, 1988.

Hrdlička, A. Growth during adult life. Proc. Am. Phil. Soc. *76:*847-897, 1936.

Hrdlička, A. Growth of the head during adult life. Further evidence. Am. J. Phys. Anthropol. *24:*127-159, 1938.

Israel, H. Continuing growth in the human cranial skeleton. Arch. Oral Biol. *13:*133-137, 1968.

Israel, H. Continuing growth in sella turcica with age. Am. J. Radiat. Ther. Nucl. Med. *108:*516-527, 1970.

Israel, H. Progressive enlargement of the vertebral body as part of the process of human skeletal aging. Aging *2:*71-79, 1973.

Israel, H. Evidence for continued apposition of adult mandibular bone from skeletized materials. J. Prosthet. Dent. *41:*101-104, 1978.

Moore, S. *Hyperostosis Cranii.* Charles C Thomas, Springfield, 1955.

Smith, R.W., Jr. and R.R. Walker. Femoral expansion in aging women: Implications for osteoporosis and fractures. Science *145:*156-157, 1964.

Trotter, M. and R.R. Peterson. Relation of transverse diameter of the adult femur to age in American Whites and Negroes. Am. J. Phys. Anthrop. *28:*65-73, 1968.

CLINICAL IMPLICATIONS OF THE AGING PROCESS

Jeffrey B. Halter

As currently conceived, there is a distinction between *gerontology*, the study of the aging process, and *geriatrics*, which is a medical specialty that is concerned with the health problems of the elderly. Geriatrics, which will be the major focus for this paper, is a relatively new and rapidly evolving discipline in the United States. Specifically, this paper will focus primarily on the impact of the growing elderly population on the medical profession.

The relative importance of geriatric medicine both now and in the future can be appreciated if one simply considers the age status of the current population and predictions of population age status for the future (Table 1). The oldest component of our society, the component made up of people over age 85, is undergoing very rapid growth in number. Indeed, although the number of older people is increasing in general, on a percentage basis, the most rapidly growing group is those over age 85 (U.S.D.H.H.S., 1987). Elderly people, particularly those over 85, are the major utilizers of our health care system; that includes the dental profession as well as the medical profession (U.S.D.H.H.S., 1987).

Approximately 12% of the population is currently over the age of 65. However, if one considers expenditure in billions of dollars for various kinds of health care services, hospitals, physicians, and long-term care facilities by age group, it is apparent that the allotment of the health care expenditures is being spent disproportionately on people in the over-65 group. For long-term care, well over 80% of the total dollars go for this age group, and that will be increasing as the elderly population increases in number. For physician's services, over 20% of the health care dollars are spent on this age group, and for hospital care it is close to 30%, even though these individuals make up only 12% of the total population. The elderly population clearly needs these services, and that need is very likely to grow as their numbers increase, particularly as the number of the very oldest of this group increases, because they tend to be the sickest. Why is that, and what are some of the health problems that they have?

Table 1. Percentage of U.S. population over the age of 65 (from Hazzard, 1983).

Year	Number (in millions)	Percent
1900	1	4
1950	12	8
1975	22	11
2000	31	12
2030	46	17

PHYSIOLOGICAL COMPETENCE IN THE ELDERLY

A notion that is currently important in geriatrics is the idea of "physiologic competence" over the life span of an individual (Hazzard, 1983). This is illustrated schematically in Figure 1. Early in life, of course, human infants are completely dependent on adults for survival; early after birth, we begin to develop physiologic competence, which continues to increase for several decades. It reaches a maximum level at early adulthood; after that peak it begins to decline. Aging could be viewed as a gradual loss of this physiologic competence. In geriatrics, and in medicine generally, we are dealing with disease processes that may accelerate this loss of physiologic competence and may be viewed as premature disease, sometimes leading to death. The difference between this normal age-related decline of physiologic competence and premature losses due to disease helps to illustrate the difference between aging and disease. In geriatrics we are dealing with people, and, in a sense, it does not really matter why they are declining; we have to address the causes of the decline and see what we can do about them. We would obviously like to prevent, as much as possible, premature adult death and disease (as we have been very successful in our society in preventing early childhood death and disease), and thereby lengthen the average life span.

A decline in physiologic competence seems to be part of the aging process, but it is a little hard to determine exactly how this comes about. There does seem to be a real association between aging and decline of physiologic function; older people just do not seem to perform quite as well in some activities as younger people, even though they may maintain health in a very rigorous way. Figure 2 shows the times for the world

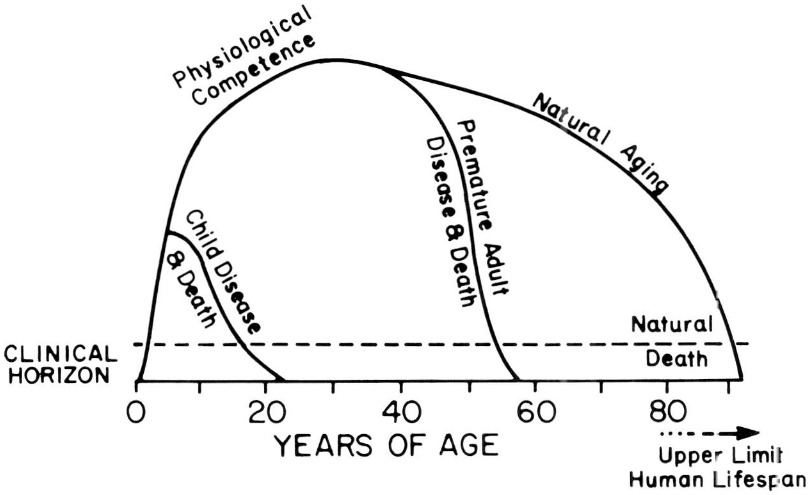

Figure 1. Causality, physiology, disease, and death across the human lifespan (redrawn from Hazzard, 1983).

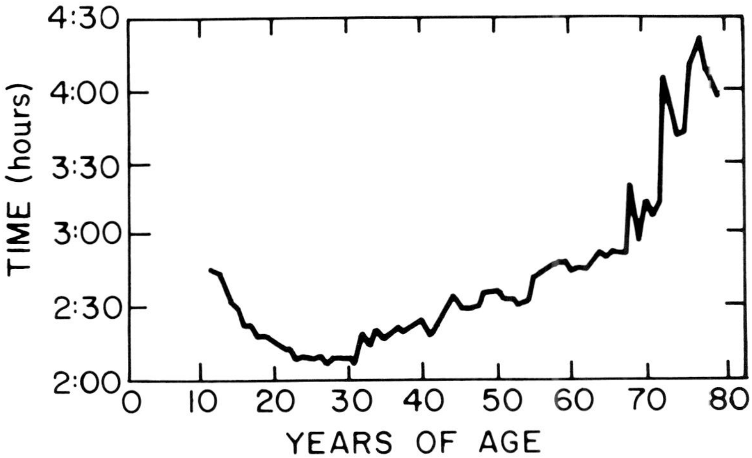

Figure 2. World marathon records for men (redrawn from Hazzard, 1983).

Table 2. The modification of aging: established aspects (from Fries and Crapo, 1981.

Aging Marker	Personal Decision(s) Required
Cardiac reserve	Exercise, nonsmoking
Dental decay	Prophylaxis, diet
Glucose tolerance	Weight control, exercise, diet
Intelligence tests	Training, practice
Memory	Training, practice
Osteoporosis	Weight-bearing exercise
Physical endurance	Exercise, weight control
Physical strength	Exercise
Pulmonary Reserve	Exercise, nonsmoking
Reaction time	Training, practice
Serum cholesterol	Diet, weight control, exercise
Social ability	Practice
Skin aging	Sun avoidance
Systolic blood pressure	Salt limitation, weight control, exercise

record for the marathon as a function of age; the lowest time is in the 20-30 age group, and there is a much longer time for people who are older (Fries, 1980). It is hard for me to accept the idea that an old person who can complete a marathon is not very fit and healthy, as healthy as an old person can probably be; yet an older person just cannot perform to the same level, in general, as a younger person. This is the purest illustration I can give (in humans) of the difference between a decline in function due to aging, which presumably this represents, versus a disease process such as coronary artery disease which would prevent a younger person from being able to perform an activity as well as a fit older person.

One of the problems that we have to deal with, which we are just beginning to address in our society, is the stereotypes that we have about older people.

VARIABILITY DURING AGING

Something that one learns in treating older people on a regular basis is that it is important to be careful about jumping to any conclusions about individuals based on their age. There is tremendous variability in the older population; it is one of the really exciting things about geriatric medicine. Young people who have a disease tend to look pretty much like the examples shown in medical textbooks, but older people do not. The appearance produced by a disease interaction in an older person may be quite different from the classic description. That makes diagnosing and treating conditions in older people challenging and interesting.

Variability is one of the important things to keep in mind in dealing with older people. Trying to determine an individual's physical or emotional condition through visual inspection alone is probably not going to provide a very accurate assessment.

Many of the physical features that are assumed to inevitably accompany old age may be modifiable. Table 2 shows a list of possible aging markers that should be or potentially could be modified. This list suggests that these factors, which are established to a certain degree, can be modified (Fries and Crapo, 1981). Many of the common problems that we associate with older people such as memory loss, osteoporosis, and skin aging could potentially be altered with the right intervention (many of these have to do with diet, exercise, appropriate dental prophylaxis) and perhaps would not then necessarily be markers of age.

"FIVE I's" OF GERIATRIC MEDICINE

In addition to the factors which may or may not be part of the aging process, there are a number of conditions that are commonly seen among elderly people that are often not addressed very well in classical medicine, but that form the basis of geriatric medicine. They are sometimes referred to as the "five I's" of geriatric medicine (Hazzard, 1983): impaired homeostasis; immobility; incompetence (referring to cognitive loss and impairment); incontinence, particularly urinary incontinence; and iatrogenic syndromes, problems resulting from interactions of patients with the health care system such as adverse drug reactions.

Impaired Homeostasis

Impaired homeostasis involves limitations of functions that maintain internal regulation, e.g., blood glucose levels and blood pressure. Our ability to function as independent organisms in an environment is dependent on our being able to regulate internal processes very tightly. To the extent that we lose the ability to fine tune or regulate our system internally, we are much less able to function as independent organisms in a somewhat hostile environment. This concept of homeostasis, which was first developed more than a century ago by the French physiologist Claude Bernard, is particularly relevant to the problems that many older people face as they lose internal homeostatic control mechanisms and consequently require a lot more structure in their environment in order to make up for those losses. Such a loss often requires that people be put into institutional settings where the environment is more controlled, which greatly cuts down the freedom of these individuals. Impaired homeostasis, therefore, is a difficult and challenging problem that many people face as they grow older.

Diabetes Mellitus. One health problem in the area of impaired homeostasis is diabetes mellitus. The highest incidence rate of new diagnosis of diabetes is in the over-age 64 group. We tend to think a lot about young people with diabetes but that incidence rate is an order of magnitude less. Estimates indicate that the prevalence of overt diabetes mellitus in people over 64 years of age is about 10% (U.S.D.H.H.S., 1987). These are not just mild abnormalities in glucose tolerance tests. This prevalence rate represents clearly abnormal glucose levels, meeting established criteria for overt diabetes. There is also evidence based on national epidemiology studies that for every person we know who has diabetes there is another person we do not know about who has it. Thus, diabetes is a very common problem among the elderly.

Blood Pressure. There are many studies that demonstrate that blood pressure increases with age in men and women. Prevalence rates of hypertension range up to 40-50% of very old populations (U.S.D.H.H.S., 1987), depending on how hypertension is defined.

Loss of Bone Mass. Women are particularly prone to develop osteoporosis, loss of bone mass, making it a very significant problem for this segment of the elderly population. There is no question that men also lose bone mass as they get older as well, so it is not a problem that is just limited to women. But the rate of loss is much greater in women, presumably due to the menopausal loss of sex hormones that are important to maintaining bone. There is also some thought that calcium balance is more negative in women younger in life, and so they tend to lose more calcium.

Immobility

We do not understand exactly why loss of bone mass is such a serious problem, but it certainly is and it both reflects and contributes to a related problem, and that is immobility. A woman who falls and breaks her wrist is not immobilized too much, although a wrist fracture can be inconvenient. A woman who falls and breaks her hip (a major group of fractures that occur in this age group), on the other hand, can experience severe limitation. In fact, there is a high mortality associated with hip fractures.

Immobility, which is common in older people for a variety of reasons related to muscle strength, balance issues and so forth, can in turn lead to falls and fractures. So there is an interrelationship here between a problem of impaired homeostasis, inability to maintain bone mass, making people very vulnerable to injury, and other changes that we see in older people that make balance and mobility limited and make them more prone to falling and injuring themselves. Very little is known about the factors that contribute to falling problems in older people. It is an area that has largely been ignored in traditional medicine, but it is getting increasing attention as this field of geriatric medicine is developing and evolving.

Incompetence

The problem of dementia, impaired cognition or mental incompetence, is a very sobering and severe problem among the elderly. The problem of dementia is not too bad in the younger old population, but when you get up to the group of individuals who are 85 years of age or older, 30% of those people have a significant problem, and in over 15% it can be classified as severe (Katzman, 1986).

There is another way to look at mental incompetence, however, that warrants emphasis. In medicine, we see the people with problems. Many people see physicians because they have a cognitive disorder and want to know what to do about it. However, the other 70% of people over age 85—those who are mentally competent—are not seen as frequently. Physicians tend to see the sick old people, particularly the older people who have dementia. Even among the aged group that is so severely afflicted with the problem, the majority of those over 65 years of age do not have this problem. It is the question of the cup being half full or half empty; one could look on the rosy side and say that 70% of people over the age of 85 do not have a severe cognitive impairment.

Urinary Incontinence

Urinary incontinence is a very common problem among the elderly, particularly in women. Men have an analogous problem, prostatic hypertrophy, which certainly can also contribute to incontinence, but the pathophysiology is completely different. Incontinence is another area that has been largely neglected by the medical profession. There is a growing body of knowledge about the causes and approaches to management of incontinence. Many patients do not even like to talk about it, and people in the medical profession do not like to ask about it because they know so little. However, when you go out into a population and specifically ask people, you find that a lot of women in the older age group have the problem of urinary incontinence.

Iatrogenic Syndromes

Drugs are being used widely for many medical reasons, and many appropriate reasons, but there is a great risk of causing problems as well. There are a number of different kinds of drug problems in the elderly: Compliance (following prescribed rules about how to use medicine) is a problem—not a problem just of older people, certainly, but it is a problem for older people because they are prescribed a lot of drugs, in general. Adverse drug reactions are very common; again, this does not seem to be particularly due to the fact that people are old. It is more due to the fact that older people are prescribed a lot of medicines, and the more medicines you have, the more likely you are to have an adverse reaction. Other problems like drug dependency and addiction also occur in the elderly; we tend to think less of that as a problem compared to a younger population, but we need to remember that older people can get addicted and have such problems as well.

In terms of some of the adverse drug reactions that older people get, there are a number of factors that seem to predispose anyone to get an adverse drug reaction. These are things you can keep in mind when prescribing medicine for people. The more drugs you have, the more likely you are to get into a problem and have a reaction. The definition of an "adverse" drug reaction is a little difficult to pin down, but it generally refers to problems like skin rashes, fevers, altered blood counts, and so forth. People who have multiple other organ system problems, particularly kidney and liver disease, are prone to develop drug problems because those are the organs that have to do with detoxifying or eliminating drugs. People with mental and cognitive problems in particular may have trouble remembering what they are supposed to do with a given medication, and use it inappropriately. People may have other kinds of impairments that may interfere with their ability to use medications correctly. Many of these disabilities are particularly common among older people.

Specifically, behavioral effects of drugs are of concern, because some older people already have cognitive or behavioral problems. One of the reasons why this is so important is because of diseases like Alzheimer's disease, about which very little can be done directly at this point. We do not know enough about Alzheimer's disease to intervene, give treatment, or reverse the process. But what can be done very effectively is to identify drugs that contribute to cognitive dysfunction in patients, and to eliminate those drugs from the treatment plan. That often can make a great deal of difference.

There are particular problems with many of the drugs that are used for central nervous system (CNS) disorders (Everitt and Avorn, 1986). Anti-anxiety agents are very commonly prescribed by both physicians and dentists. In an office setting, there is a certain amount one can do to control patient anxiety just by creating a relaxing environment and having the right professional manner. However, sometimes it is necessary to administer a drug to try to put a patient at ease so that the physician or dentist can work effectively. The principle that must be kept in mind is that use of an anti-anxiety agent poses a risk, particularly among older people.

ECONOMICS OF GERIATRIC MEDICINE

In medicine there is an ongoing discussion of various kinds of interventions for various conditions and their cost-benefit ratio. Ultimately, what is a benefit? Some people try to define benefit in terms of specific economic values: is it worth spending $2,000 to fix a child's jaw so that the teeth are in better shape later in life? You know what the cost is; what is the potential benefit? If an individual has an estimated economic "value" of $170,000, maybe it is not so bad to invest $2,000 in him Is it worth spending $2,000 on an 85-year-old's jaw to make her more functional? It is unlikely that such a person will earn any more money or contribute to the gross national product. However, perhaps if the jaw

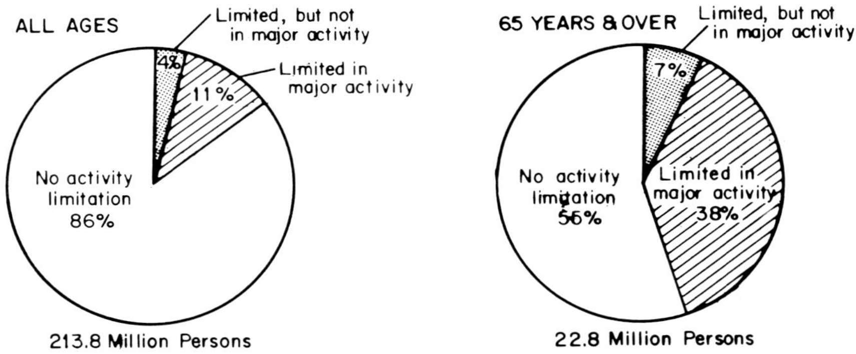

Figure 3. Percent of the elderly with activity limitation due to chronic conditions, United States, 1978, excluding individuals in institutions. Percents may not add to 100 due to rounding. (Redrawn from National Center for Health Statistics, 1983.)

is fixed she will be able to eat better; if she eats better, perhaps she will not lose weight, have negative nitrogen balance, lose muscle mass, become infirm, and end up in a nursing home. Thus, an individual's capacity for creating wealth should not be the only criterion upon which to judge the benefit of a medical or dental intervention.

Another way of looking at the issue of the cup being partially full or partially empty is shown in Figure 3. This is a plot of the percentage of elderly people with activity limitations due to chronic conditions; there are many such people in the United States. On the other hand, the majority of older people do not have such limitations. Limitations can also be environmental. When my father lived in Minneapolis, his activities were limited in the winter just because of the climate. He moved to California and he is a lot more active than he used to be, because the environment is conducive to activity. Again, in medical practice we tend to see the older people who have activity limitations, and not those people who are more active and functional.

A vicious circle can occur in the elderly because of the relationship between an individual's physical health, mental health, and social situation. People who have health problems lose their ability to function, cannot interact with society as much, and have to be protected; they can become socially isolated. As a result of that isolation, they are subject to malnutrition and neglect, which can lead to weakness, make them prone to accidents and infection, necessitate confinement to bed, and increase vulnerability to physical illness, thus fueling the cycle with more disability. There are situations in which people with one or two disabilities can continue to function relatively well for a time. However, eventually an individual is no longer able to compensate, and the vicious cycle of conditions develops. For those in health care professions who deal with older people, this situation is like trying to maintain a leaking dike during a flood. The first hole appears in the area of economic or social supports, so you try to plug that; then a medical problem creates another hole and sets the cycle off again. It may require considerable time and effort by multiple health care professionals to try to address the problems of a person who gets into this situation.

We use the concept of geriatric assessment, which focuses on the functional status of individuals, for this process (Rubenstein, 1987). This approach is less disease-oriented than traditional medicine, and it takes several domains into account: the physical domain (the traditional side of medical care), the psychological domain, and the socioeconomic domain, which traditionally has not been part of medicine. If you focus on just one of these domains alone, you will have many problems dealing with the functional limitations of elderly people. The concept of a multidisciplinary geriatric team has grown out of this need for comprehensive assessment. It has been demonstrated to have utility in dealing with a number of health problems of the elderly population. The team should include individuals who have expertise in dealing with physical problems, psychological problems, and social problems. To the extent that we can, we have tried to make sure that dentists are included in such a team. We would like to see that expand in the future, because we feel that part of the overall problem with many individuals has to do with nutritional support at home, and dentists have a very important role in that regard.

Many exciting things are happening in the field of geriatrics, at least within medicine. I hope analogous development will occur in the field of geriatric dentistry. We have a great deal to offer the many older people who are active and want to stay that way. I believe that we can also do a lot to improve the quality of life for the older people who have the misfortune to be in poor health, and who need our attention.

REFERENCES

Everitt, D.E. and J. Avorn. Drug prescribing for the elderly. Arch. Int. Med. *146:*2393-2396, 1986.

Fries, J.F. Aging, natural health, and the compression of morbidity. N. Engl. J. Med. *303:*130-135, 1980.

Fries, J.F. and L.M. Crapo. *Vitality and Aging: Implications of the Rectangular Curve.* W.H. Freeman, San Francisco, 1981.

Hazzard, W.R. Clinical rationales for the inclusion of geriatrics in medical education. In: *Proceedings of the Regional Institutes of Geriatrics and Medical Education.* Assoc. Am. Med. Coll., Washington, D.C., 1983.

Katzman, R. Alzheimer's disease. N. Engl. J. Med. *314:*15, 1986.

National Center for Health Statistics. *Changing Mortality Patterns, Health Service Utilization, and Health Care Expenditures, 1978-2003.* Vital and Health Statistics, Series 3, Number 23. D.H.H.S. Publ. No. (P.H.S.)83-1407, Hyattsville, 1983.

Rubenstein, L.Z. Geriatric assessment: An overview of its impacts. Clin. Ger. Med. *3:*1-15, 1987.

U.S. Department of Health and Human Services. *Personnel for Health Needs of the Elderly through Year 2020.* N.I.H. National Institute on Aging Administrative Document, Bethesda, 1987.

THE CONSEQUENCES OF ADULT CRANIOFACIAL GROWTH

Rolf G. Behrents

Lulled by a feeling that all that is necessary to know about the adult craniofacial complex is already known, one might easily ask why developing a new perspective on growth-related change in the adult craniofacial skeleton is an important endeavor for the orthodontist. The answer is clear; with the ever-increasing number of adults seeking orthodontic treatment, it becomes imperative that we generate an awareness and understanding of the age-related conditions associated with the adult. It is important to do so because general *concepts* of adult craniofacial growth determine how we *think* about individual adult patients, and *knowledge of the events* of craniofacial growth determine how we *treat* these patients.

It is necessary, therefore, that we re-examine the stereotypes that have evolved concerning growth and aging in the adult craniofacial complex. In the past, many published accounts regarding adult orthodontic treatment were negative. Caution and even avoidance of adult orthodontic therapy were recommended (Vanarsdall and Musich, 1985). For example, in 1901 MacDowell wrote:

> Impossible age. After the age of 16 years, a complete and permanent change in transition of the occlusion, the author believes to be almost impossible. There may be a case or two in rare exceptions, but as a rule the change cannot be accomplished successfully owing to the development of the adult glenoid fossa and the density of the bones and muscles of mastication.

Despite a major reorientation of orthodontics toward adult patients during the past decade, many of the mental limitations of the past are reflected in the current literature. For example, Vanarsdall and Musich (1985) suggested that mechanical options are limited in the adult because of lack of a neuromuscular adaptability, a much narrower range of TMJ adaptability, cessation of growth, an increased susceptibility to bone loss, and slower tooth movement. Such statements are made in spite of the fact that little research has been conducted to substantiate negative assumptions about the potential for successful orthodontic treatment in adults. Research has been narrowly focused on the child and adolescent; very little research has been conducted on the adult. We now treat more adults than in the past but continue to be limited by a stereotypic attitude about them; seldom do we consider the biological possibilities for adults. We think and talk of life as if it were comprised of a series of chapters in a book: prenatal, neonatal, childhood, adolescence, young adulthood, middle age, old age, etc. But these stages are artificial; life is a continuous series of events, each blending from and into the next. As a case in point, there is a rational basis for believing that adults *grow*.

A BIOLOGICAL BASIS FOR GROWTH IN ADULTHOOD

Focusing exclusively on the periods of life where rapid and obvious change occurs is too restrictive, since it is known in many disciplines that developmental processes remain intact and that changes in morphology continue long after puberty. Outward changes of adult aging are often noted, generally in regard to superficial appearance and function, but these changes also have a biological basis at the cellular, tissue, organ, and systemic levels. Many studies have been carried out to document the physiological and morphological aspects of aging (Andrew, 1971; Finch and Hayflick, 1977; Sinclair, 1978; Kohn, 1978; Behrents, 1984, 1985*a,b,c*), and it is clear that change occurs on all levels, continually, during the adult period. Since the overall bodily changes involve many different tissues, including bone, and numerous biochemical mechanisms, it should not be surprising that alterations can occur at the osteological level, and even to the extent that morphological changes can be recorded.

In addition to constant remodeling of bone through resorption and deposition, other gross changes are noted with regard to age in the adult. Enlow (1982) has pointed to a change in the width of bone cortex with age. He has also suggested that there is an increase in the width of various canals and cancellous spaces of bone in the aged as the result of osteoporosis. This aspect of bone development, or bone redistribution, involving gross changes on both periosteal and endosteal surfaces has been extensively studied by Garn. His studies have demonstrated that up through the fourth decade, continuing bone gain occurs in both sexes by means of subperiosteal deposition and endosteal deposition, resulting in an increase in cortical thickness and a maximum bone mass between 30 and 40 years of age (Garn, 1970, 1972, 1981). Thereafter, and throughout life, subperiosteal apposition and endosteal resorption result in increased external dimensions (more for females) and an expansion of the medullary cavity. These two effects result in a decrease in cortical thickness with age, but increased bone diameters.

This generalized remodeling of bones along with increases in bone diameters (periosteal and endosteal) due to continued remodeling has been reported consistently in the literature for the rib (Epker and Frost, 1965; Epker *et al.,* 1965; Sedlin *et al.,* 1963), femur (Smith and Walker, 1964; Trotter *et al.,* 1960; Ruff and Hayes, 1982; Smith and Frame, 1967), second metacarpal (Garn *et al.,* 1967; Garn *et al.,* 1968), humerus (Pfieffer, 1980), tibia (Garn, 1970), vertebrae (Ericksen, 1976; 1978), and skull (Israel, 1973). These studies generally included both males and females ranging in age from the fourth through the ninth decade (Garn, 1983). What is clear from this research is that bone is somewhat unique among connective tissues: it is continuously remodeled, irrespective of physiological demand or aging.

A PERSPECTIVE ON ADULT CRANIOFACIAL GROWTH

During the adult period, with the panoply of biological changes occurring in general and with osteologic changes in particular, it is only logical to expect that whole osteological systems, like the craniofacial complex, might be altered as part of the usual aging process. According to Enlow (1981), once basic adult form is obtained, gross (not histologic) remodeling is static unless there is an alteration of the environment such as a change of function, a change in biomechanical circumstance, loss of teeth, etc. However, he has also shown that such environmental changes are quite likely, indeed certain (Enlow, 1981). As a demonstration of this effect, Enlow and co-workers (1976) found that extensive remodeling occurs throughout all mandibular areas after dental loss.

Even with all the available evidence indicating that bones can and do become altered throughout life, it has generally been accepted that the craniofacial complex does not change to any appreciable, practical, measurable extent during adulthood. This notion has been accepted in the absence of substantiation. On the contrary, however, there is evidence that the craniofacial complex does indeed *grow* during adulthood. Many studies have attempted to document such change, but the work of investigators who have had the opportunity to study longitudinal material probably reflects the most important aspects of current views about adult craniofacial growth.

Studies by Buchi (1950), Thompson and Kendrick (1964), and Kendrick and Risinger (1967) document that facial dimensions increase with age. Perhaps the most convincing evidence for continued growth of the head, however, has been provided by Israel. In a series of investigations (1967, 1968, 1971, 1973, 1977), utilizing both cross-sectional and longitudinal material, Israel came to the conclusion that the cranial skeleton and vertebrae generally increased in all dimensions studied. From this, he inferred that a process of virtually symmetrical magnification was occurring, on the order of 1% per decade.

Israel's work did not go unchallenged. Tallgren's (1974) studies showed no consistent growth-related change in the adult craniofacial skeleton, leading her to suggest that Israel's findings could be accounted for by errors in technique. On the other hand, Forsberg (1976, 1979) examined individuals in their twenties and concluded that craniofacial change continued into the thirties. Similar conclusions were reached by Hunter (1966), Cleven (1969), Susanne (1977), and Sarnas and Solow (1980).

Bolton-Brush Longitudinal Study

An extensive longitudinal study was recently conducted (Behrents, 1984, 1985*a,b*) as an extension of the Bolton-Brush Growth Studies in order to investigate further the growth-related changes that take place in the aging craniofacial skeleton. The Bolton-Brush Growth Studies were extensive longitudinal growth investigations conducted in the 1930s and 1940s, spanning the period from birth to young adulthood. A total of 113 of the original participants were recalled for the collection of new (older) adult data. Together with existing records, 163 cases spanning ages 17-83 years (524 lateral cephalograms) were utilized to determine the nature and extent of any adult craniofacial alterations. The orthodontically untreated portion of the sample consisted of 113 individuals, 90 of whom possessed a full complement of teeth at the time of recall. It should be noted that this longitudinal sample of adult material is one of the largest ever collected. The Bolton Standards are based on 32 individuals (Broadbent *et al.,* 1975), while the Michigan Standards are based on 83 individuals (Riolo *et al.,* 1974).

The results were surprising and unequivocal: adults continue to grow. This was evident in nearly all portions of the craniofacial complex, the

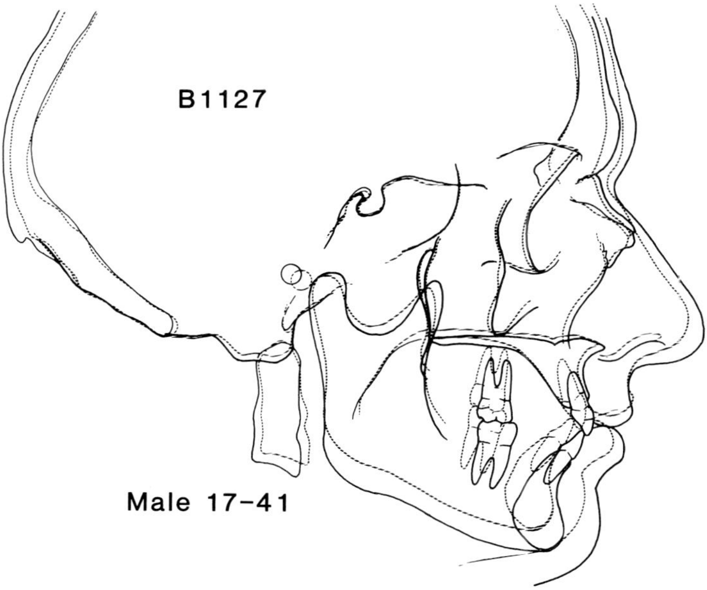

Figure 1. Superimposition: untreated male. Dashed lines indicate the initial tracing.

vertebrae, and the bones of the hand. After adjusting the cephalometric data for magnification, analysis revealed continuing growth of the craniofacial complex throughout all age levels that is similar to typical adolescent alterations but of lesser magnitude and rate. Growth in adulthood was the rule, not the exception; over 100 individuals of the possible 113 (untreated sample) demonstrated significant growth alterations during adulthood.

Changes in both the size and shape were noted for a number of areas of the face. In young adulthood, the direction of craniofacial growth was specific to the individual's growth pattern; i.e., "horizontal growers" grew horizontally and "vertical growers" grew vertically. However, in later adulthood, vertical dimensional changes appeared to be common to all adults. Older adults were less protrusive, with a flattening of the facial profile, and had longer facial heights. Craniocervical and vertebral changes were also encountered (Figs. 1, 2).

Definite differences in the nature and extent of some changes in craniofacial growth were found between males and females. Typically, the craniofacial skeleton in females was smaller and grew less in adult-

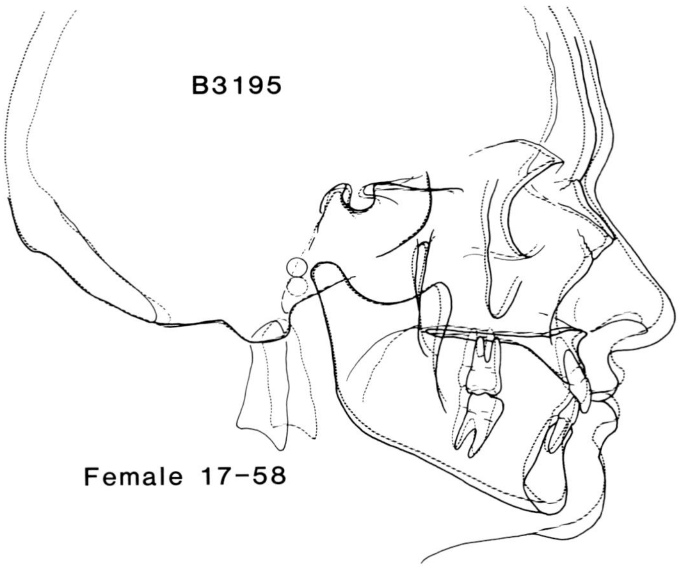

Figure 2. Superimposition: untreated female. Dashed lines indicate the initial tracing.

hood. Craniofacial growth in females was expressed more vertically than in males. In the male, a forward (counterclockwise) rotation of the mandible was typical, while in the female, a backward (clockwise) rotation was common. Beyond this, sexually dimorphic features were particularly evident in the orbital region, which were more related to the orbit itself than to the glabellar region (Figs. 3, 4). Data further suggest that females undergo a generalized growth deceleration in late adolescence, as do males, but that females uniquely exhibit a reacceleration of growth in later years (Figs. 5, 6).

Dental changes were considerable and consistent with the osseous changes. In both sexes, the maxillary incisors became more upright, but only in the females was there evidence that the lower incisors became more protrusive. Molar adjustments, coincident with mandibular plane alterations, were present and differed for each sex, the upper molar tilted forward and the lower molar became more upright in the male. The converse occurred in the female (Figs. 7, 8).

Soft-tissue changes were more dramatic than skeletal alterations, but remained concordant with the skeletal change. The nose became more

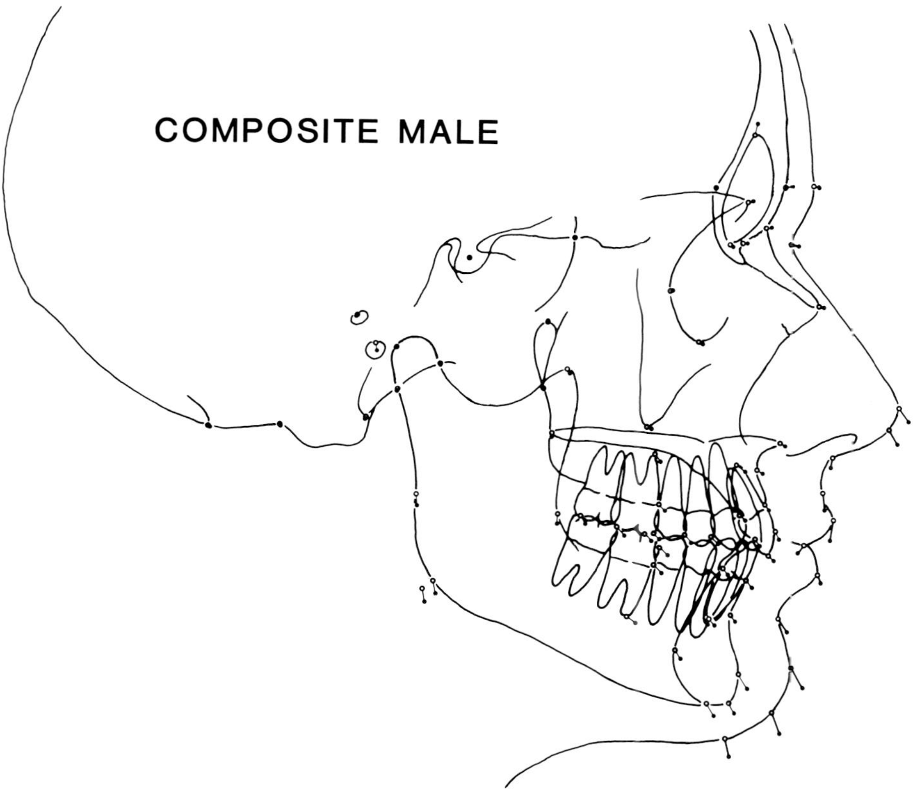

Figure 3. Composite male constructed on the basis of mean locations of landmarks oriented to sella-nasion and registered at sella. Regional anatomy is added to the initial landmark locations (open circles). Closed circles denote the final landmark locations. Reprinted from Behrents, 1985*a*.

prominent and the tip became located more inferiorly. The lips became less prominent and became located more inferiorly with age as the face lengthened and flattened. This resulted in a very distinctive decrease in the nasolabial angle.

Summary: Craniofacial Growth in the Adult

Based on our biases and supported by the literature, we have assumed that growth ceases in adulthood because it slows dramatically following puberty. Available evidence now documents that adults continue to grow

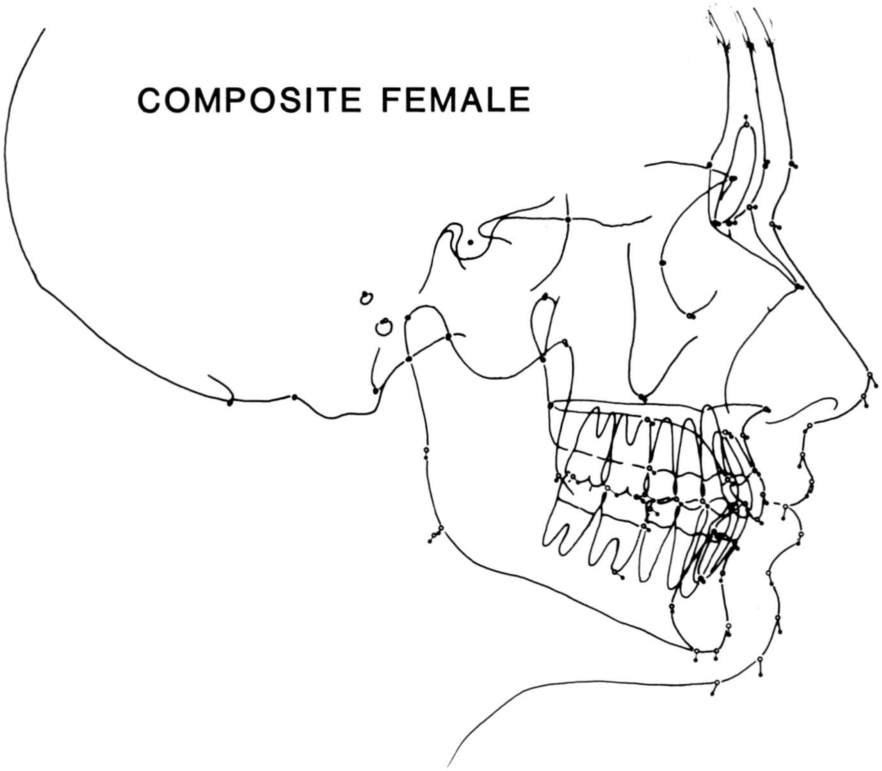

Figure 4. Composite female constructed on the basis of mean locations of landmarks oriented to sella-nasion and registered at sella. Regional anatomy is added to the initial landmark locations (open circles). Closed circles denote the final landmark locations. Reprinted from Behrents, 1985*a*.

into the later stages of life and that such growth is different for the two sexes. This conclusion is clearly supported by the recent results of the Bolton-Brush Longitudinal Growth Study reported above. Moreover, this conclusion is supported by other previous longitudinal studies and, in addition, generally support the findings of adolescent studies conducted by Subtelny (1959), Chaconas (1969), Wei (1969), Chaconas and Bartroff (1975), Ingerslev and Solow (1975), Bibby (1979), and Bishara and Jakobsen (1985).

The amount of change that occurs in the adult craniofacial skeleton per year is very small compared to the dramatic increases noted in child-

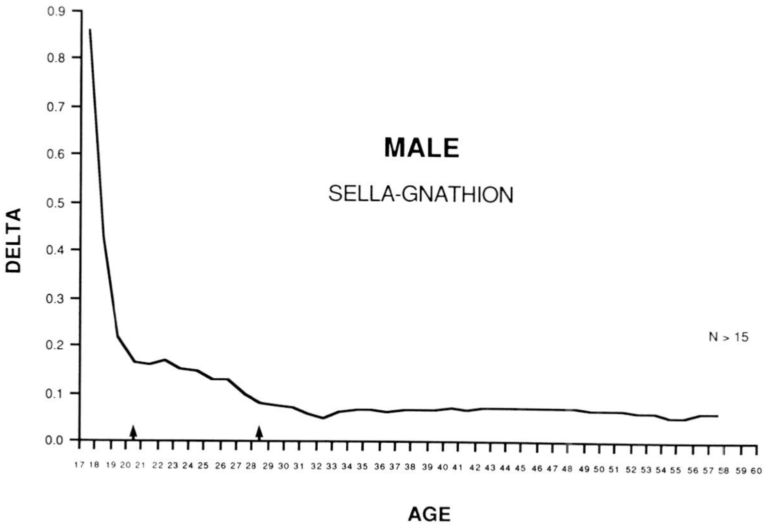

Figure 5. Growth deltas for the measure sella-gnathion in the male. While the individual deltas for each year are small, their cumulative effect may have a significant bearing on a change in dimension for an individual. Mean deltas were calculated by partitioning the individual deltas across age.

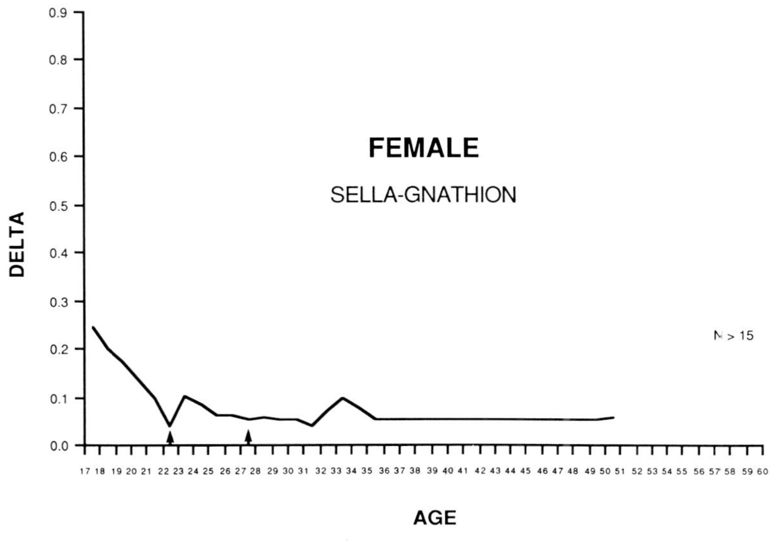

Figure 6. Growth deltas for the measure sella-gnathion in the female. While the individual deltas for each year are small, their cumulative effect may have a significant bearing on a change in dimension for an individual. Mean deltas were calculated by partitioning the individual deltas across age.

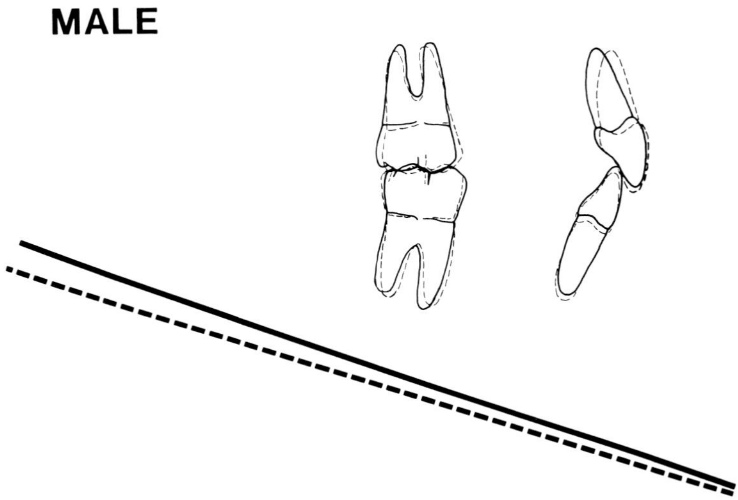

Figure 7. Dental changes in the male. Dashed lines indicate the final positions of the teeth and the mandibular plane. Reprinted from Behrents, 1985*a*.

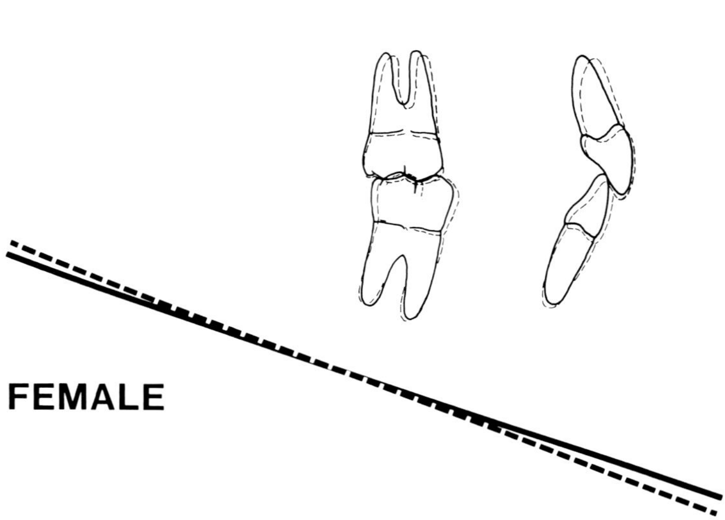

Figure 8. Dental changes in the female. Dashed lines indicate the final positions of the teeth and the mandibular plane. Reprinted from Behrents, 1985*a*.

hood and adolescence, but it is nonetheless important. It is important because growth per unit time has no major significance, whether in childhood, adolescence, or adulthood. It is the cumulative effects of the growth processes that are important. In adulthood, a 2-10% change can be noted which, over time, can have a substantive effect on the jaw relations and a larger relative effect on the positions of teeth. Compare this to a typical cumulative change of 1.5 mm involved in correction of a Class II malocclusion to a Class I. So, within an arch that measures 60 mm from front to back, a 2.5% change has occurred. Given that this 2.5% change is considered significant to the clinician, a 2-10% change in the adult craniofacial skeleton might result in an equal or greater alteration, especially if the growth is poor in nature.

Given that such adult growth can be demonstrated, an important question arises: how can this information be used to understand, control, and predict the outcome of treatment? To address this question, several related investigations have been conducted with intention of subjecting the notion of adult growth to the test of usefulness, and identifying potential consequences of its application. In other words, might such information on adult growth be used beneficially to treat adults, or might it be used to help treat adolescents, and might such information be used to justify inappropriate treatments? Based on these considerations, the remainder of this paper will explore three general areas of consequence related to adult craniofacial growth: diagnosis, treatment, and post-treatment changes.

CLINICAL CONSEQUENCES: DIAGNOSIS AND TREATMENT PLANNING

Knowledge of the biological potential of the patient, whether child, adolescent, or adult, provides the conceptual framework for all diagnostic and treatment-related procedures. It is anticipated, therefore, that the knowledge that the adult patient is capable of growth will have an immediate impact on diagnostic procedures. Specifically, a thorough understanding of the potential for growth in the adult patient is necessary before a thorough understanding of treatment is possible, before treatment outcomes can be predicted, before growth can be controlled, and before maximum potentialities can be realized.

It must be understood that craniofacial growth in the adult will alter, in large measure, the final morphological and functional patterns of dental and associated skeletal relationships throughout life (Schudy, 1974). The all too common conceptual view that adults are characterized by a static dentition and craniofacial skeleton is likely to mislead clinicians, encouraging negative or pessimistic views of treatment outcomes in adults and restricting thoughtful analysis of adult treatment.

Besides the conceptual importance of this notion, its impact on diagnosis and treatment planning has more direct effects on two commonplace manipulations. First, when standards are used to compare individuals to norms it is necessary, just as it is in adolescence, to reference appropriate age and sex norms for, in this case, the adult. This has been recognized before (e.g., Goldsman, 1959; Christie, 1977). For example, it would be unwise to assess a 40-year-old male using a currently available 18-year-old standard. A practitioner doing so might mistake normal vertical changes involving the chin as excessive facial height requiring a reduction genioplasty. The demonstration of change in adulthood requires that age-appropriate standards be used to assess the adult; few such adult standards exist. Second, acknowledgement that adults continue to grow renders growth predictions as arbitrary, incomplete, and further flawed. If growth forecasts are to be improved, then new information on the adult will have to be included.

In addition, a myriad of simple answers to important treatment planning questions will have to be determined. For example, where should one position the teeth proportional to age and consistent to the changed soft tissue? Where is the smile line in the adult? The naturally occurring maxillary incisor uprighting means that it is necessary to determine the proper torque for these teeth in the adult. When extractions are necessary, should second bicuspids be elected more than first bicuspids so that the already straightened profile is not compromised? And, how should one arrange the teeth in order to maintain consistency with TMJ adjustments and growth yet to come? New planning parameters will have to be determined.

CLINICAL CONSEQUENCES: TREATMENT

The typical amount of adult growth described above, i.e., 2-10%, will have little effect on standard orthodontic treatments. The increments of growth occurring on a yearly basis are, in most individuals, small and usually will neither help nor hinder the progress of a typical two-year treatment. This applies to the standard treatments with fixed appliances and applies with emphasis to the use of removable appliances. Evidence of adult growth should in no way be used as a rationale for the utilization of functional appliances in the adult; results of such attempts will be lengthy and discouraging (for further clarification, see Behrents, 1984). This has been shown quite clearly by McNamara (1983). However, there are other aspects of treatment where knowledge of craniofacial growth in adults will provide benefits.

Adjustments of the Occlusion

Even small incremental changes will have an effect on procedures where the amount of change produced through treatment is itself very small. This applies directly to procedures which are designed to adjust the occlusion. Where the removal of microns of enamel constitute the extent of the treatment, age-related changes in the skeleton and dentition will likely adjust the occlusion to a greater extent. Thus, the most meticulously performed occlusal adjustment should not be considered final; additional procedures may be necessary at later times. A major adjustment such as an orthodontic adjustment of the occlusion also should not be considered final; later readjustments may also be necessary due to the growth of the craniofacial complex (Bandeen and Timm, 1985).

Treatment of the Class II Adolescent

Attempts have been made to determine whether the information gained from the adult study described above has application to adolescent treatment (e.g., Johnston, 1986; Pool, 1987). Conventional clinical wisdom suggests that certain types of orthodontic correction are not affected by the sex or age of the patient (i.e., sex and age as variables that affect the response of a patient to treatment are typically ignored) in spite of numerous reports indicating that male and female craniofacial configurations are different (Hellman, 1932; 1935; 1940; Wei, 1969; Ingerslev and Solow, 1975; Hunter and Garn, 1981; Enlow, 1982). In addition, it was clear from the adult recall data (Behrents, 1984, 1985*a,* 1985*b*) that males and females differ in growth and development. Further, it was speculated that females with Class II malocclusions, once treated, might be more prone to sagittal relapse after treatment because of the predisposition in females for a clockwise rotation of the mandible with age and time.

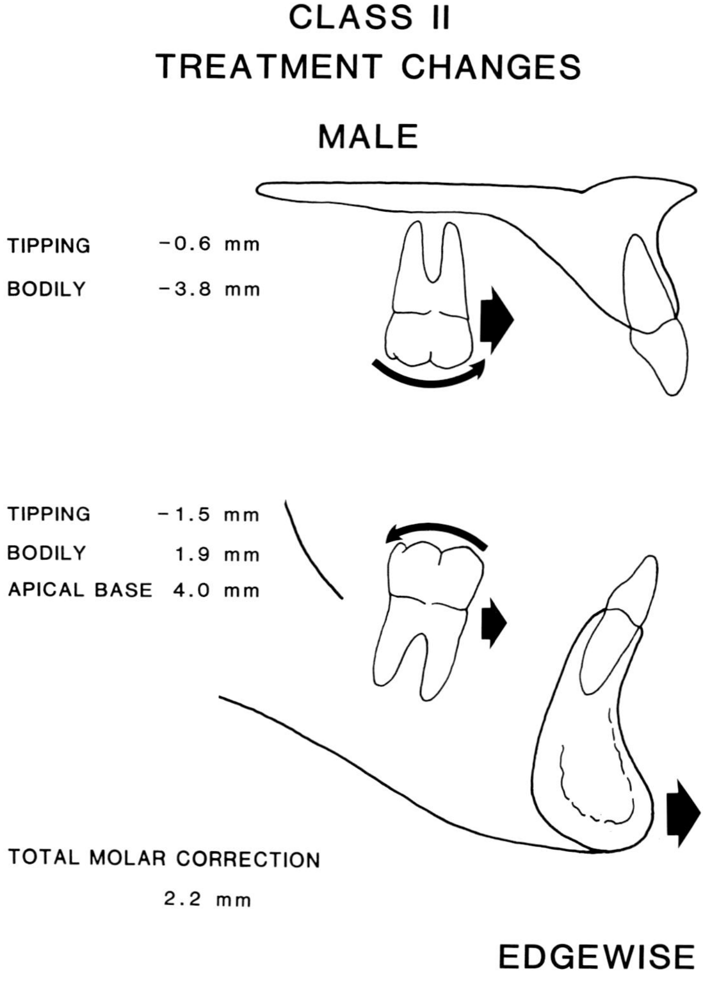

Figure 9. Treatment changes during Class II correction in the male. Bodily movement of the molar correction. Positive values indicate factors which favor a Class II correction while negative values work against a Class II correction. From Pool, 1987.

Such speculation led Pool (1987) to investigate the relative contributions of sex and age to the correction of the Class II situation (36 males and 54 females treated with standard edgewise mechanotherapy, beginning at approximately age 13). Using the analysis developed by Johns-

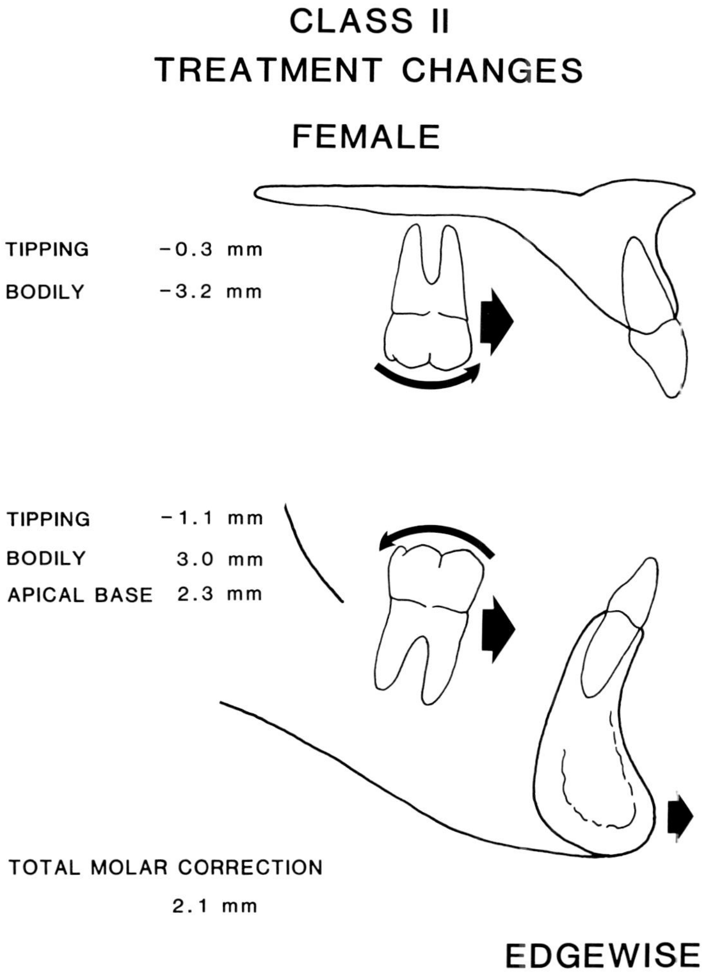

Figure 10. Treatment changes during Class II correction in the female. Bodily movement of the molars plus the apical base change sums to equal the total molar correction. Positive values indicate factors which favor a Class II correction while negative values work against a Class II correction. From Pool, 1987.

ton (1986), which seeks to assess the contributions of a number of factors in their relative contribution to the overall correction, Pool was not able to draw conclusions regarding the relationship of tooth movement to age; however, this was accomplished elsewhere. Johnston (1986) showed that in the correction of an adolescent's Class II malocclusion, bodily movement of teeth in conjunction with sagittal growth alterations are the major contributors; tipping of teeth plays a minor role. In the older patient, with growth not contributing as strongly, in addition to bodily movement, more tipping of teeth is required to effect the correction.

Pool did uncover some interesting aspects of the effect of sex on the correction of Class II malocclusions. In males, Class II correction depended more on an apical base change (e.g., growth); in females, Class II correction depended more on mesial movement of the lower molar along with a small apical base change (Figs. 9, 10). In large measure, the growth of males accomplishes the correction, whereas with females, tooth movement is necessary. Translated into patient management terms, it is indeed fortunate that females are generally more cooperative in treatment procedures, for they require more precise tooth movement, more headgear wear to restrict maxillary growth, and they are more prone to relapse because their Class II configuration and subsequent growth are not favorable; Class II females are difficult cases to treat and require more skill on the part of the operator and more cooperation on the part of the female patient. On the other hand, a "normal" Class II male literally grows into a large portion of the correction, perhaps even assisted by augmented mandibular growth in late adolescence (Harrison, 1986; Kemp, 1986; Johnston, 1986); cooperation is less critical in the male, and that is indeed fortunate.

It is speculated that in the correction of a Class III malocclusion, males would be difficult to treat, cooperation would be more critical, and relapse would be more likely. Because of the tendency for a clockwise rotation of the mandible in females, treatment would be aided by growth, cooperation would be less critical, and relapse would tend to favor the maintenance of correction.

Timing of Orthognathic Surgery

Another aspect of treatment which is directly affected by awareness of the potential for adult growth involves the determination of the appropriate time for performing orthognathic surgery (Behrents and Harris, 1986). Apparently there is no specific, absolute age that is ideal for surgery to correct craniofacial deformities. However, a commonly held notion is that, where possible, surgery should be delayed until growth has ceased so as to diminish the opportunity for relapse associated with

Table 1. Number of individuals who gained or lost in ray 2 bone dimensions as measured from the younger to the older age.

Bone	Pooled Sample		Males		Females	
	Gained	Lost	Gained	Lost	Gained	Lost
Distal	33	3	24	3	9	0
Middle	32	4	24	3	8	1
Proximal	25	12	21	7	4	5
Metacarpal	0	37	0	28	0	9

Two bones (distal and middle) for one male were not available on both films and thus are missing data points.

growth. It is generally believed that growth usually ceases between 16 and 18 years of age in males and somewhat earlier in females, usually between 14 and 16 years of age.

Studies used to establish these guidelines usually have centered on the growth and development of a variety of complex body systems. Emphasis has been given to the assessment of height, weight, somatotype, dental status, and skeletal maturation of the vertebrae, hand, and craniofacial region among others. The assessment of maturity of the bones of the hand and wrist is currently the most popular method of timing of facial surgery.

Radiographic analysis of bones of the hand and wrist is typically used to determine somatic and craniofacial maturity milestones (Fishman, 1982; 1987; Hägg and Taranger, 1980; 1982). Unfortunately, while answers to specific questions are sought through analysis of such data (correlation of event to event), only general answers can be provided. It may be that the maturation of the bones of the hand and wrist is an imperfect method for forecasting craniofacial events. In addition, since continuing growth of the craniofacial complex has been demonstrated even into the later stages of adulthood (Behrents, 1984), a fact which seriously undermines the value of using hand-wrist radiographs to determine when craniofacial growth "has ceased," it is necessary to re-examine this method to determine if a practical alternative can be located.

Garn and co-workers (1972) have reported standards for metacarpal and phalangeal lengths for the bones of the hand for both sexes from infancy through adulthood. All persons older than 18 years of age were considered to be adults; this group consisted primarily of the parents of the child participants. It is interesting to note that the mean values for the second metacarpal of the adult were lower than the values for 18-year-olds, which may be a result of sampling or secular trend. This finding, however, was not borne out in a recent study by Behrents and Harris (1987). A longitudinal analysis of 37 individuals followed by means of matched pairs of standardized hand-wrist radiographs from young adulthood (minimum of 19 years of age; mean = 22 years) to later adulthood (mean = 54 years) demonstrated that the lengths of the distal and middle phalanges (and proximal phalanges in the male) continue to increase in overall length while the metacarpals significantly *decrease* in size (mean = 2.1 mm). This was interpreted as another example of differential, continuing, adult morphological alteration in a complex system; it is also clear that the nature and directions of change differ in the head and the hand (Table 1).

In essence, the head continues to grow in adults, and assessments of the maturation of the hand as presently performed may not be as useful as indicators of craniofacial maturity as has been thought. Consequently, in cases where growth of the patient is considered an important factor in the timing of surgery, the issue of identifying the optimal age must be addressed.

In response to this need, data were scrutinized to form generalized growth curves for males and females during adulthood (Behrents, 1984). This analysis showed, in general, that growth proceeds in a decelerating fashion throughout adulthood with a variance that is attenuated with time. These investigations suggest that if growth is a major factor in the timing of surgery and relapse due to growth is to be minimized, the best method to evaluate the relative slowing of craniofacial growth would be to follow a patient over time into his or her mid-twenties, using periodic cephalograms. This would provide information on the magnitude and timing of growth in that individual. In the absence of this individual patient evaluation, an alternate method based on correlating skeletal behavior with chronological age would suggest that surgery be performed after the age of 21, when growth increments per year have generally plateaued with minimal future deviation in the magnitude of growth for both sexes. If the procedure can be delayed even further, it would be appropriate to perform surgery after age 28, when variability is minimized (arrows in Figs. 5 and 6).

In predicting the outcome of a surgical procedure, one must account for as many of the sources of variability as possible. In this account, two sources of variability are discussed: surgical treatment and growth. Re-

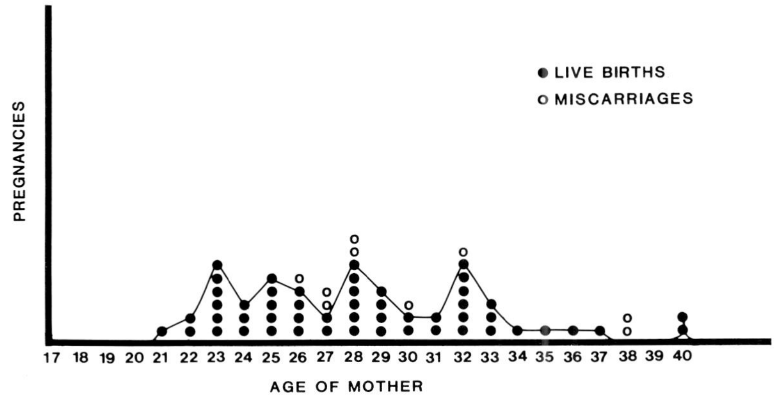

Figure 11. Occurrence of pregnancies in the female sample of Behrents, 1984.

gardless of the timing of treatment, the variability introduced by surgery remains a factor in the predicted outcome. The variability associated with adult growth cannot be eliminated through knowledge of adult growth characteristics, but it *can* be reduced. Further, based on these same guidelines, "early" child or adolescent surgery might be expected to be a very unstable endeavor (Gibson, 1987).

Sexual Dimorphism

The growth curves presented for male and female adults (Figs. 5, 6) are not identical. While the male curve suggests a general deceleration in growth, the female curve is erratic, with a deceleration in the late teens and oscillating activity in the twenties and thirties (Fig. 6).

Supplemental data collected on females was scrutinized to assess the difference between males and females. One subjective correlation emerged: it appeared that the re-acceleration of growth activity related (slightly out of phase) to the condition of pregnancy (Fig. 11). The reason for this might be relatively simple. An embryo is not structurally or functionally capable of growing itself. The pituitary gland is not formed and growth hormone is thus not present until the end of the second month *in utero*. Further, it is known that, for a time, control of the processes involved in embryonic growth is supplied by the pituitary gland of the mother and only subsequently is relegated to the placental tissues. If the mother is controlling the growth of the embryo and if the mother is receptive to her own system, then she may grow herself.

While entirely speculative when first presented, there is evidence that the scenario of increased maternal skeletal growth during pregnancy may be sound. First, it is clear that hormones which control or modify growth are available at all ages, and that new controls are possible during pregnancy in particular (Gregerman and Bierman, 1974). Furthermore, in human pregnancy, calcium is accumulated, apparently in preparation for lactation. Obviously such an accumulation potentially could affect the skeletal tissue. There are several reports of increased skeletal size and/or density associated with pregnancy in humans (Smith, 1967; Garn, 1970). Garn (1970) suggested that during pregnancy, bone is deposited periosteally and endosteally, while during lactation, bone is lost on corticoendosteal and endosteal surfaces, though very little bone is lost on the periosteal surface. This two-stage process results in increased bone diameters.

Collectively, these data suggest that there are changes in skeletal metabolism and remodeling during pregnancy. Miller and co-workers (1986) demonstrated this quite clearly. Their data indicate that maternal skeletal growth peaks between early- and mid-pregnancy and appears related to coincidental increases in the placental lactogens (chorionic somatotrophins) and somatomedin.

The direct application of the apparent stimulation of bone growth during pregnancy to the clinical arena is unclear at this point; no practical treatment regimen is immediately apparent. It is clear, however, that there would be both appropriate and inappropriate applications for such knowledge, if it proves correct. It is also intriguing to speculate whether stimulation of bone growth during pregnancy, if established, might have some impact on the structures of the temporomandibular joint and might be related to the increased prevalence of dysfunction seen in females during the third and fourth decades of life. Moreover, it is possible that such a resumption of growth activity might affect the stability of results of previous orthodontic and orthognathic treatments. Further work in this highly speculative area is needed.

CLINICAL CONSEQUENCES: POST-TREATMENT

Perhaps the greatest consequence of adult growth relates to the post-treatment period. Schudy (1974) suggested that growth can have far-reaching effects on the dentition of individuals who have completed orthodontic therapy in terms of alignment of the lower anterior teeth, overbite maintenance, and temporomandibular joint-occlusal harmony. He states that "Knowledge of this final segment of growth is, therefore, crucial to successful and comprehensive treatment of the growing child and should be of concern to all orthodontists."

Relapse

Long-term stability of the treated case has been an area of concern for almost as long as correction of malocclusion has been performed. Unfortunately, little progress is noted in the orthodontic and orthognathic literature over the years regarding solving this universal problem. Instead, it is continually suggested that a correct diagnosis and treatment plan, followed by the application of skilled mechanotherapy designed to place teeth in certain axial, arch, and osseous positions, and then followed by stabilization of the treatment result, will minimize or eliminate the potential for undesirable post-treatment tooth movement. Clinicians tend to assume a finality of result in the well-treated case. This perception is supported by the tendency for those cases considered by both clinician and patient to be failures to tend to go away, physically and mentally; practitioners seem not to be tremendously concerned by their attrition, since they usually have ample evidence of success at hand. Nevertheless, relapse is still a considerable problem which is encountered in each case to a greater or lesser extent.

A number of factors have been investigated in an attempt to elucidate their role in relapse following treatment of a malocclusion. The orthodontic profession has sought the "initiator," laws (i.e., 100% of variability explained), and axioms (i.e., series of rules) for guidance in dealing with relapse. Key topics for consideration have included arch form alteration, occlusion, positions of the teeth, third molars, supporting tissue reorganization, latent growth, muscle function, amount and direction of correction, and several other factors. Unfortunately, even though a number of theories, opinions, and axioms regarding treatment have been developed, neither time nor research have provided solutions to the problem of post-treatment instability. In this area, one possible etiologic factor which has not been adequately explored is post-treatment growth.

Incisor Irregularity. Little and co-workers (1981) documented a number of dental changes that might be expected following treatment. In terms of causation, a number of authors have suggested numerous treat-

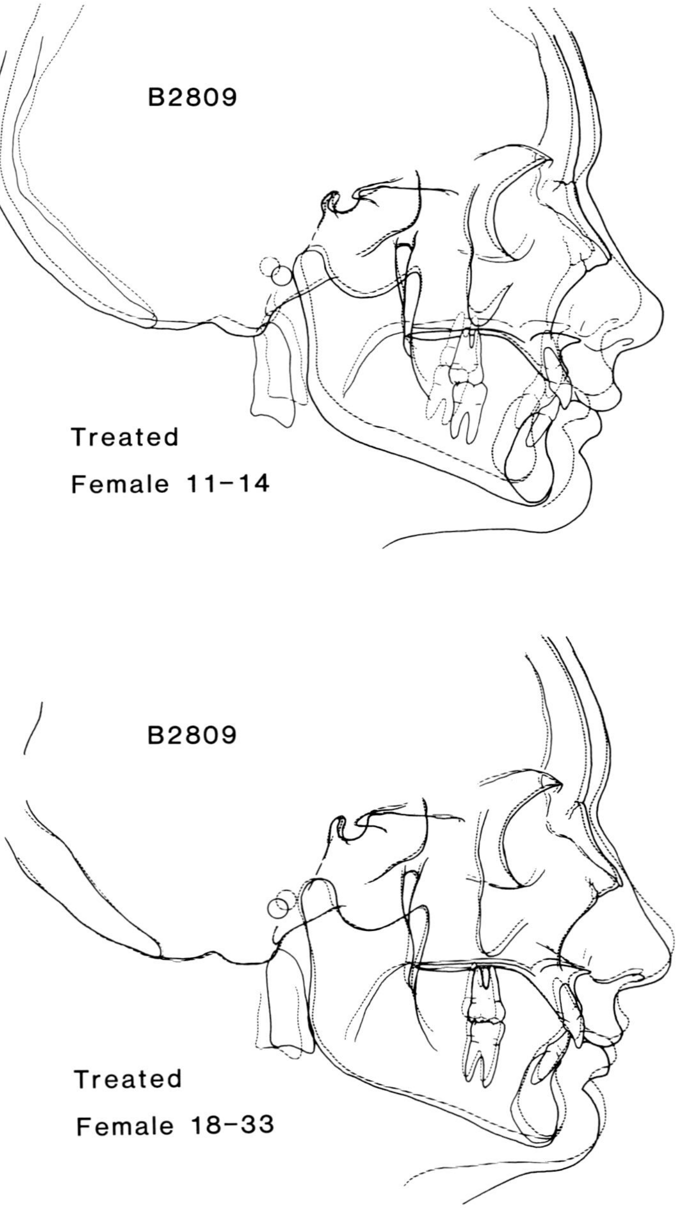

Figure 12. Female patient who initially demonstrated a Class II malocclusion, was treated and retained (upper), but grew out of the correction (lower).

ment attributes and naturally-occurring factors as possible causes of incisor irregularity. Expansion and later decreases of arch form, failure to upright the incisors over basal bone, improper crown and root angulations and inclinations, pressure from erupting third molars, mesial drift, and unanticipated mandibular growth pushing against the maxillary incisors, thus forcing the mandibular incisors lingually, have all been implicated as factors directly contributing to lower incisor irregularity.

The investigations of Carmen (1978) and Kapley (1982) took a different direction. They investigated the factors contributing to mandibular anterior dental crowding in untreated individuals, and found that incisor irregularity may become more or *less* given time. In an attempt to account for this variability, many dental and skeletal relationships were investigated to determine possible correlations. While no definitive associations were found, it was generally apparent that anatomic factors tended to predispose an individual to crowding or lack of crowding, while dental factors tended to determine the severity of the crowding (slight crowding or very crowded).

Recently, Williams (1985) studied the long-term stability of the dental arch after treatment. His conclusions were both expected and unexpected. Even though the cases were well treated, one-third of the crowding returned. Specifically, Williams found that: (1) intercanine widths narrowed to values smaller than those seen pretreatment; (2) the longer the period of retention, the less severe the post-treatment crowding; (3) the longer the period after retention ceases, the greater the crowding; (4) growth of the craniofacial skeleton continued through the oldest age studied (22 years); and (5) the greater the post-treatment change in the growth of the maxilla, the greater the *regularity* of the lower anterior teeth ($p < 0.08$). Treatment positions (cuspid width, molar width, incisor inclinations, etc.) were not important in explaining irregularity; rather, it appears that growth is the important factor in terms of post-treatment stability. This finding is consistent with the findings of Behrents (1984, 1985*a,b*), which demonstrated that the maxilla continued to move forward with time as the upper incisors uprighted. The results collectively suggest that the key to understanding relapse of the lower incisors may involve understanding the growth of the maxilla and the uprighting of the maxillary incisors. Mandibular growth and the positions of the lower incisors would play a secondary role in this process.

Sagittal Relapse. Compared with incisor irregularity, relapse of sagittal corrections (Class I reverting back to the original Class II or Class III relationship) has received far less attention in the literature. One must, therefore, assume that this condition occurs with far less frequency than incisor irregularity. However, if this type of relapse does occur, retreatment regimens are usually very involved and time-consuming for the patient and the practitioner. Thus, such relapse is considered a significant problem.

Growth that occurs after treatment can have a tremendous impact on the sagittal relationship of the corrected case, and can even have an impact on a person who has not been treated such that they grow into a treatable condition. What is important to realize with regard to examples of continuing bone alteration in the adult is that it continues. Further, bone alteration continues in spite of attempts at alteration through various short-term treatments. Figure 12 shows a patient who grew (poorly) before orthodontic treatment, was treated, and then literally "grew" into a relapsed condition during adulthood. It must be stated that in this example, treatment was effective in reducing the asymmetry, but not in ceasing biological alteration to a pattern consistent with prior performance. This agrees with studies by Bishara and Jakobsen (1985), who found that facial configuration in untreated individuals was maintained up to age 25, and the comments of Schudy (1974), who feels that orthodontic treatment does not change the basic character of growth of the craniofacial complex. It should be obvious that clinicians who assume that the state achieved at the end of treatment is a "final" result are incorrect.

That growth plays a major role in sagittal relapse was demonstrated quite clearly by Kemp (1986). Aided by the cephalometric analysis developed by Johnston (1986), which generally is used to determine the relative contributions of a number of factors to an overall correction, Kemp sought to determine the relative contributions of a number of factors to an overall "uncorrection" (i.e., relapse). In his study on 71 treated individuals (previously Class I and Class II) who were recalled several years after retention was complete, both dental arch relapse and sagittal relapse were noted. He found that correction of a Class II malocclusion resulted from movement of the lower molars (1/3 more than Class I) and a favorable apical base change (more than Class I cases). Together, these factors overcame unfavorable movement of the upper molars. In retention, cases that were previously Class II stayed corrected by means of a favorable apical base change due to the fact that these cases exhibited approximately three times more forward relative horizontal growth of

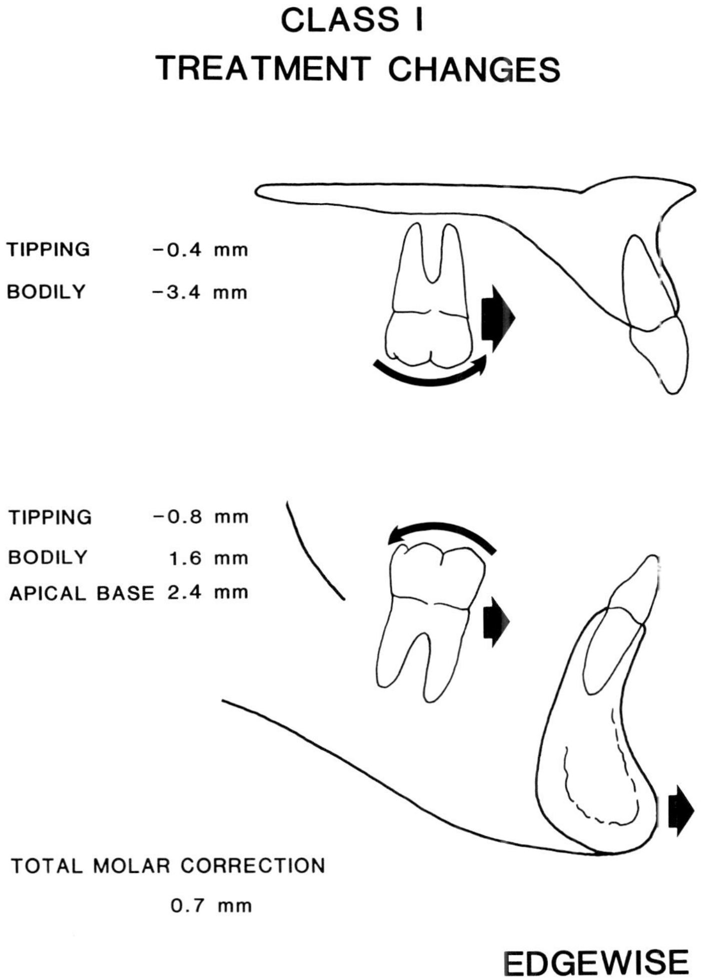

Figure 13. Treatment changes during Class I correction. Bodily movement of the molar correction. Positive values indicate factors which favor a Class I correction while negative values work against a Class I correction. From Kemp, 1986.

the mandible compared to that seen in Class I cases; maxillary and mandibular tooth movements favored relapse (Figs. 13-16). This agrees with Harrison (1986), who noted that untreated Class II individuals, especially males, showed some potential for extra "catch-up" growth in their teens.

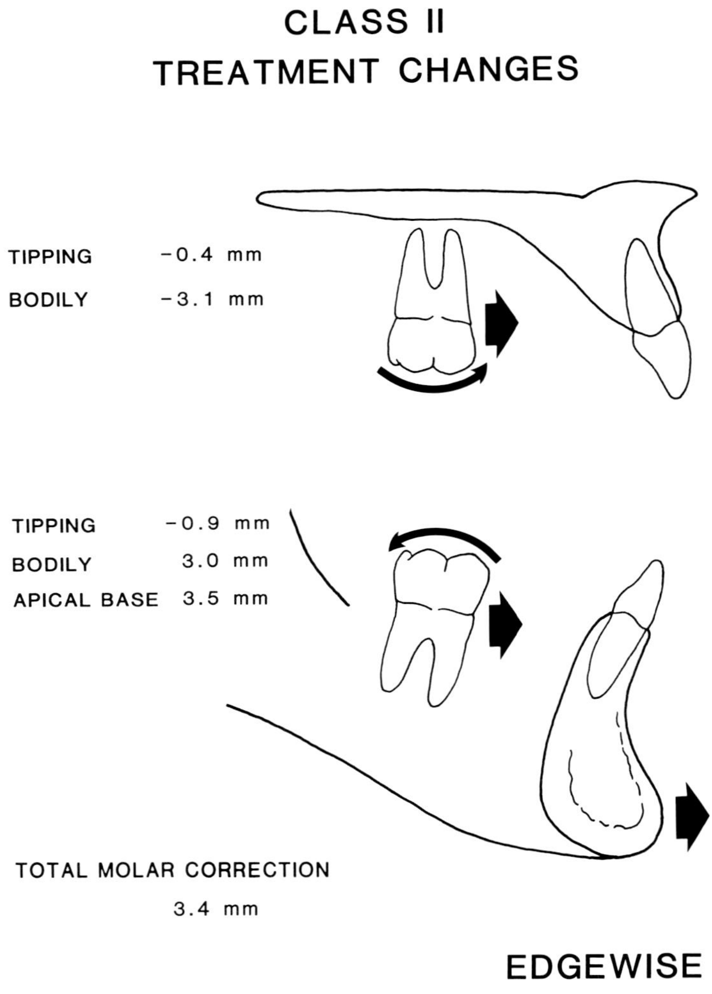

Figure 14. Treatment changes during Class II correction. Bodily movement of the molars plus the apical base change sums to equal the total molar correction. Positive values indicate factors which favor a Class II correction while negative values work against a Class II correction. From Kemp, 1986.

These results indicate that the forward growth of the mandible is the main factor involved in maintaining a Class I molar relationship post-treatment in the Class II cases: i.e., growth maintains the correction. It was also shown quite convincingly that patients with poor growth patterns,

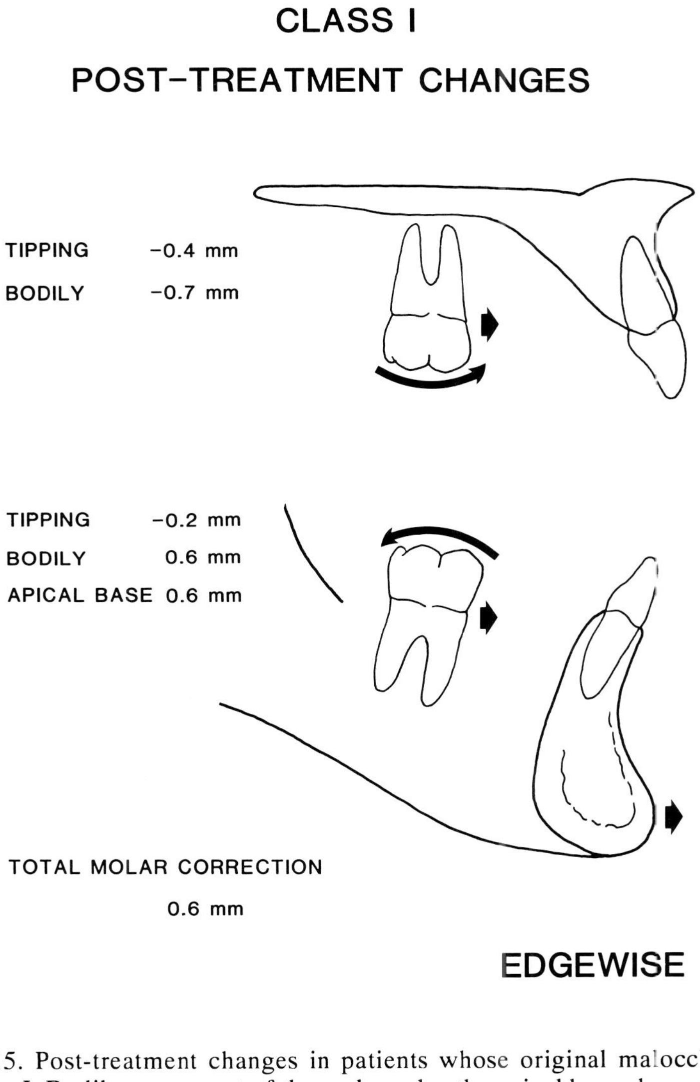

Figure 15. Post-treatment changes in patients whose original malocclusion was Class I. Bodily movement of the molars plus the apical base change sums to equal the total molar correction. Positive values indicate factors that favor maintenance of the Class I correction while negative values work against maintenance of the Class I correction. From Kemp, 1986.

in this case, small horizontal change, are most likely to experience relapse of the sagittal relationship. Thus, placing a Class II molar relationship into a Class I apparently had a beneficial effect on growth.

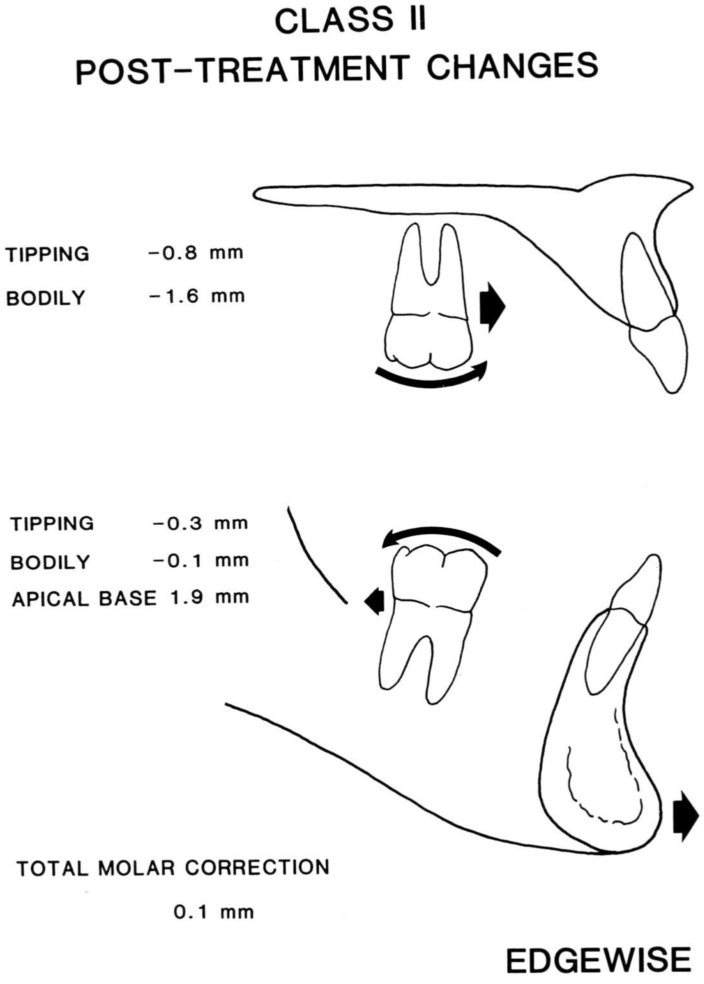

Figure 16. Post-treatment changes in patients whose original malocclusion was Class II. Bodily movement of the molars plus the apical base change sums to equal the total molar correction. Positive values indicate factors which favor maintenance of the Class I correction while negative values work against maintenance of the Class I correction back toward the original Class II malocclusion. From Kemp, 1986.

This latter finding has bearing on a study of untreated adult individuals (sample from Behrents, 1984) recently completed by Harris and Behrents (1988). Dental casts were measured in order to assess the relative stability of various molar relationships between younger adulthood (average age = 20 years) and older ages (average age = 55 years). This was done to determine whether a Class I molar relationship is stable, thus making it a primary treatment objective. In this longitudinal assessment, it was found that Class I relationships were 100% stable in all of the 69 cases. In contrast, Class II relationships became significantly worse by becoming more Class II ($\bar{x}$ = 0.8 mm); no case spontaneously reverted to a Class I occlusion. Class III cases became more Class III with time ($\bar{x}$ = 1.2 mm), with only one case in 13 improving spontaneously. These findings are in agreement with Williams (1971), who found no evidence to support the assumption that good mandibular growth in a child will correct a Class II relationship spontaneously without treatment.

Taken together, the findings of Williams (1985), Kemp (1986), and Harris and Behrents (1988) tend to indicate that incisor relapse is related to maxillary changes, while sagittal relapse is related to mandibular changes. Further, the attainment and maintenance of a Class I molar relationship will likely be more stable as a result of subsequent growth, making it a desirable treatment objective.

Further, the findings of Behrents (1984, 1985*a,b*) and Johnston (1986) demonstrate that an untreated sagittal problem (Class II or III) is likely to persist and eventually worsen, leading to continued dentoalveolar compensation. This process appears to occur whether or not growth is favorable (Hixon and Klein, 1972; Solow, 1980). But when a sagittal condition is treated to a Class I molar relationship by whatever manner of appliance, growth is favored, and the result is likely to be relatively stable. On the other hand, regardless of the prior manner and type of mechanotherapy, poor growth after treatment will cause relapse of the sagittal condition. Unfortunately, the variability is considerable, and one does not know what to expect.

Retention

Given the above findings, the present state of our knowledge is still not adequate to support any assumptions about the stability of sagittal corrections. Until this void is bridged, important questions regarding retention will remain unanswered. One simple, but necessary, question involves the duration of retention procedures. Given the fact that adults continue to grow and taking into account the notion that they can grow

Table 2. How long should the case be retained?

Empirically Derived Guidelines
1. "...answer varies from not at all to forever."
2. "...as long as the patient is interested in his teeth."
3. "...as long as the patient will wear it (retainer)."
4. "...until the musculature reaches a condition of balance with the dentition."
5. "...18 months."
6. "...until the problem of the third molars has been resolved."
7. "...7 years if the case is finished at 13-14 years of age.
8. "...for as short a period of time as possible."
9. "...as long as one possibly can."
10. "...for at least as long as active treatment."
11. "...as long as patients will allow."
12. "...until they go away to college."
13. "...play it by ear."
14. (for children) "...until they become adults."
15. (for adults) "...indefinitely."
16. "...forever."
17. "...as long as five years after the removal of tooth-removing appliances."

References available on request.

Table 3. What determines how long the case should be retained?

1. The original malocclusion
2. The distance the teeth have been moved
3. The state of the development of the teeth
4. Which teeth were moved
5. The type of movement
6. The correctness of the diagnosis
7. The correctness of the final tooth position
8. The presence of expansion
9. The interdigitation
10. Whether the patient is growing
11. The morphology of the teeth
12. The age of the patient
13. What the patient expects
14. What the parent expects
15. What the orthodontist expects
16. The type of treatment (extraction or non-extraction)
17. Which teeth were removed
18. The sex of the patient

References available on request.

poorly, how should retention of correction be achieved, and for what period should the procedure be continued?

Procedures. Given the above findings, it is clear that where growth disturbances were present before treatment, some consideration should be given to retaining the correction by means of appropriate appliances. In other words, the typical maxillary Hawley appliance and mandibular fixed appliance seem inadequate to retain a Class II correction. While these appliances are appropriate to address concerns of dental irregularity, they do not address the previous growth problem. It seems prudent, therefore, to prescribe the wearing of a functional appliance or a headgear to maintain the correction of a previous sagittal problem. This is also the contention of Graber (1966), Muchnic (1970), Nemeth and Isaacson (1974), and others.

Duration. In terms of standard retention procedures designed to maintain stability of the teeth and the sagittal correction, it is often suggested that a careful examination of the original malocclusion and the treatment result may provide valuable guidance in determining the best method of retention for each case. But, even with careful individualized post-treatment diagnosis and retention planning and the utmost care, it is still difficult to determine how long retention procedures should be continued.

Most often, the duration of retention seems to be determined empirically (Table 2). In general, the more severe the original case, the longer the period recommended (Table 3). For adults, the retention period suggested is often stated in indefinite terms. This is ironic, for after adolescent orthodontic treatment is completed and the patient becomes an adult, practitioners tend to assume a cessation of the processes of osseous and dental change and retention is terminated. On the other hand, after adult orthodontic treatment is completed, practitioners tend to assume that the processes of osseous and dental change can continue, and retention is maintained indefinitely. Both situations involve adults, with one considered stable and one not.

Unfortunately, only a relatively few studies have been performed to establish a biological basis for determining the appropriate duration of retention (e.g., Barrow and White, 1952; Moorrees, 1959; Hotz, 1966; Edwards, 1968; Reitan, 1967, 1969; Gallerano, 1976). Studies directed at the questions of reorganization of supporting tissue or of transverse dimensional changes of the dental arches indicate that a minimum of two years in retention is necessary. But this guideline does not address reten-

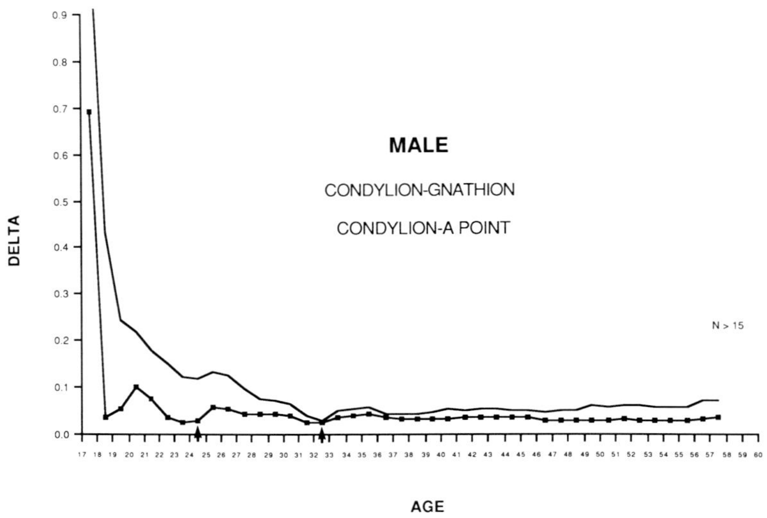

Figure 17. Maxillary and mandibular adjustments in untreated males.

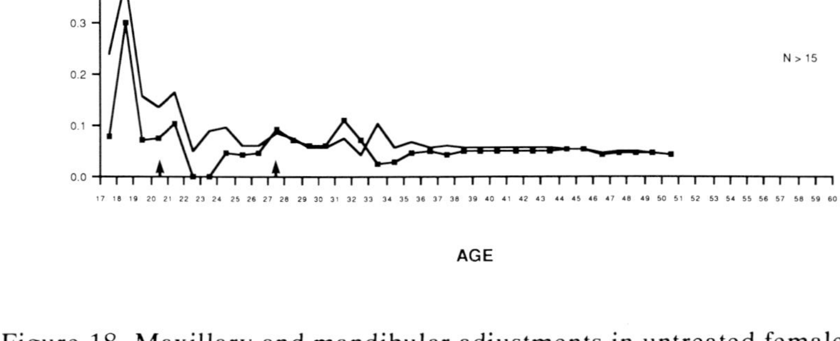

Figure 18. Maxillary and mandibular adjustments in untreated females.

tion with respect to the growth adjustments that can occur after treatment.

It is the contention here that the teeth will not be stable until the bones and soft tissue are, and that the best that can be hoped for is *relative* stability. For ultimate stability the length of the period of retention should be indefinite for both the adolescent and the adult. As a general treatment policy, however, this attitude is not practical. As an alternative, guidelines such as the following might prove useful. For males, based on the level of growth activity and the maxillomandibular adjustments that occur, retention into the mid-twenties is suggested; for females, retention until the early twenties seems appropriate (Figs. 17, 18). There is also some evidence to suggest that retention might be prudent during pregnancy. Further, in certain types of cases, other retention parameters seem appropriate because of the activity of the mandibular and occlusal planes: the Class II (treated) female and the Class III (treated) male seem more prone to relapse. The duration of the period for applying retention should be lengthened in these cases.

Third Molars

Traditionally, third molars have been held in low esteem. They are often considered vestigial organs which are absent, malformed, or for which there is no room. More often than not, it is assumed that third molars will impact and will have to be removed. Removal is usually justified by clinicians on the basis of preventing pathological sequelae and because of the supposed (but not documented) eruptive and disruptive effect of third molars on the integrity of the dental arch. Further, it is suggested that such extractions be conducted earlier, rather than later, in order to avoid the increased incidence of surgical complications seen in adulthood. Orthodontists, oral surgeons, and general dentists are relatively quick to decide that third molars must be removed.

In the current literature, the assumption that third molars will impact (especially if poorly angulated) and, therefore, require extraction remains the predominant theme (Bishara and Andreason, 1983; Bishara and Burkey, 1986; Johnson and Quirk, 1987; Tullock and Antczak-Bouckoms, 1987). Haas (1986) suggested that "dentistry's general low regard for third molars will dictate their removal when any aberrancy exists." Bishara and Andreason (1983) echo this sentiment, suggesting that even when third molars are asymptomatic and free of pathosis, their removal may be justified simply on the basis of impaction or malposition.

On the other hand, third molars are occasionally considered a valued commodity to be used as reserves for transplants, as abutments in a mutilated dentition, and as potentially useful functional contributors to the occlusion. As a result, several prediction schemes have been developed to determine whether or not third molars will ultimately erupt.

It is currently believed that third molars fail to erupt mainly due to a lack of available space. Given that it has been demonstrated that continued growth of the craniofacial complex occurs (Behrents, 1984, 1985*a,b*), however, it is possible that sufficient space might be developed in adulthood to allow eruption. This is not taken into account by current prediction methods. In fact, when the X-rays of the Behrents (1984) sample were viewed to determine what had occurred with regard to the third molars (third molar removal was not as commonplace in the 1930s and 1940s as it is today), it was found that in a surprising number of cases, third molars erupted successfully during adulthood. This seriously undermines the value of growth predictions that purport to be 90% accurate even at the early age of 8 years, but do not take into account adult growth.

Prediction. Several prediction schemes, most of which are based on an assessment of retromolar space, are available to foretell the eruption of third molars. In order to assess the efficiency of several prediction schemes in view of this new information on adults, a sample of cephalometric films was selected for study. Two groups were analyzed: films of 14-year-olds who had all four third molars impacted, as verified on adult films (minimum of 56 years of age) and a group of films of 14-year-olds in whom all four third molars ultimately erupted into occlusion. All films (15 males and 8 females) were randomized and subjected to various prediction schemes outlined in the literature (Leydard, 1953; Turley and Chaconas, 1975; Schulhof, 1976; Ricketts, *et al.,* 1976; Ricketts, 1979) and non-prediction biases. In addition, the films were shown to graduate students and faculty members who, without the aid of any measurements, were asked to guess whether the third molars would erupt or impact; this survey was termed the "Wisdom Test."

As can be seen in Table 4, the Turley method (Turley and Chaconas, 1975) was 100% correct *if its instructions were followed;* those molars predicted to impact, if removed, of course would not have erupted, and those predicted to erupt, erupted. Unfortunately, in several cases the disaster of removing teeth which ultimately would have erupted would have occurred. Nonetheless, the Turley method was the most efficient overall

Table 4. Efficiency of prediction of third molar eruption. The sample was selected on the basis that all third molars were present in adulthood. This included both impacted (9) and erupted conditions (14). The sample included 15 males and 8 females.

Method	Overall Prediction Efficiency	Prediction of Impaction	Prediction of Eruption
Turley	15/23 (65%)	9/9 (100%)	6/14 (43%)
Leydard	9/23 (39%)	9/9 (100%)	0/14 (0%)
"Wisdom Test"*	307/506 (61%)	133/198 (67%)	174/308 (56%)
(a) Non-prediction	9/23 (39%)	9/9 (100%)	0/14 (0%)
(b) Non-prediction	14/23 (61%)	0/9 (0%)	14/14 (100%)

*The "Wisdom Test" involved merely showing each one of the films to faculty and students (22 judges) and asking whether the third molars will erupt or will not erupt. This "eyeball" technique is commonly employed in terms of the reasoned uncertainty involved in orthodontic decision-making.

Non-predictions:

(a) "all third molars will impact" is a pessimistic bias.

(b) "all third molars will erupt" is an optimistic bias.

Table 5. Deficiency of prediction of third molar eruption. The sample was selected on the basis that all third molars were present in adulthood. This included both the impacted (9) and erupted conditions (14). The sample included 15 males and 8 females.

Method	Overall Prediction Efficiency	Prediction of Impaction	Prediction of Eruption
Turley	8/23 (35%)	0/9 (0%)	8/14 (57%)
Leydard	14/23 (61%)	0/9 (0%)	14/14 (100%)
"Wisdom Test"	199/506 (39%)	65/198 (33%)	134/308 (44%)
(a) Non-prediction	14/23 (61%)	0/9 (0%)	14/14 (100%)
(b) Non-prediction	9/23 (39%)	9/9 (100%)	0/14 (0%)

(65%). However, it is perhaps more important to observe the results of these analyses in terms of their "wrongness" instead of "rightness" (Table 5). In viewing Table 5, it is clear that mistakes are made in 35% of the decisions utilizing the Turley method while 39% of the "guesses" involved in the Wisdom Test and the non-prediction of "all will erupt" were nearly as good. Still, focusing on the deficiency of each method is not the best perspective as the two wrong guesses do not carry equal consequences. Prediction of impaction, and extracting the third molars when they would have erupted if preserved, is a disaster with perhaps life-long consequences. On the other hand, when the third molars actually become impacted it is an inconvenient but correctable situation; the impacted teeth can still be extracted. More conservative estimations of eruption produce an equal number or fewer consequential errors than the Turley and Leydard methods (Table 6). It is clear that the Leydard technique is heavily biased toward extraction, as is the non-prediction of "all will impact." It is clear that the two relatively undesirable outcomes outweigh any advantage given by the prediction schemes. The Turley method (if its advice were followed) would lead to routine enucleation (germectomy). Further, the Turley method never achieved the 90% accuracy claimed. This finding corroborates the work of Fink (1976), who found the Turley method to be 49.5% correct overall, and also found its accuracy to decrease in direct proportion to the length of the prediction interval.

The Wisdom Test, which performed relatively well, is an example of the structured uncertainty which is commonly applied in orthodontic diagnosis. Utilizing this technique, the prognosticator would know the possible future states, but not the exact probability associated with each. This analysis also demonstrates that the decision maker is not ignorant, as is often assumed by various prediction schemes; in fact, the practitioner uses knowledge of nature and empirical clinical experience, which often have a conservative practical bias.

Any prediction scheme must be assessed on its ability to cause benefit as well as its ability to cause harm. On the basis of the above discussion, it would appear that the decision to treat (extract) is easily made and the decision is correct the majority of the time. But such a decision to treat also implies responsibility if the decision is wrong; at this point in time, a conservative approach to prediction seems warranted, especially when ethical concerns are included.

Because it was apparent that the Wisdom Test was somewhat successful in determining which third molars would erupt or impact, two subsequent studies were conducted utilizing a broad approach to prediction that involves many aspects of craniofacial configuration instead of focusing on measuring and predicting the retromolar space. Goggans

Table 6. Assessment of regrettable, uncorrectable decisions during predictions of third molar eruption. The sample was selected on the basis that all third molars were present in adulthood. This included both impacted (9) and erupted conditions (14). The sample included 15 males and 8 females. The column on the far right is the most telling.

Method	Overall Prediction Disasters	Prediction of Impaction	Prediction of Eruption
Turley	8/23 (35%)	0/9 (0%)	8/14 (57%)
Leydard	14/23 (61%)	0/9 (0%)	14/14 (100%)
"Wisdom Test"	134/506 (26%)	0/198 (33%)	134/308 (44%)
(a) Non-prediction	14/23 (61%)	0/9 (0%)	14/14 (100%)
(b) Non-prediction	0/23 (0%)	0/9 (100%)	0/14 (0%)

(1986) studied a sample of 48 individuals evenly divided between sexes and eruption patterns. Longitudinal data were collected from cephalometric films at 9, 11, 13, 15, and 17 years of age. Primarily on the basis of the works of Hellman (1936, 1938) and measures used in contemporary prediction schemes, he analyzed 106 variables at each age and performed inferential testing to determine the significant differences between those individuals with erupted third molars and those with third molars impacted. Goggans found that many variables were important across age, and relationships conducive to third molar eruption were different for males and females.

Encouraged by these findings, Kincaid (1986) attempted to validate the findings of Goggans and to develop a new prediction scheme by selecting an additional sample of 13-year-old patients (N = 50), performing a stepwise discriminant function analysis on the Goggans data, and by determining the prediction efficiency of the selected variables by predicting eruption status of the original sample (N = 48) and the new sample (N = 50). The stepwise discriminant function selected 13 variables for the female and six for the male. When tested against the original sample (N = 48), prediction efficiency was 100% for both sexes. However, when tested against the new comparable sample (N = 50), prediction efficiency diminished. In males, the six variables predicted impaction correctly 58% of the time and predicted eruption correctly 64% of the time. For females, the scheme predicted impactions correctly 25% of the time, and eruptions 91% of the time. Obviously this prediction scheme was incon-

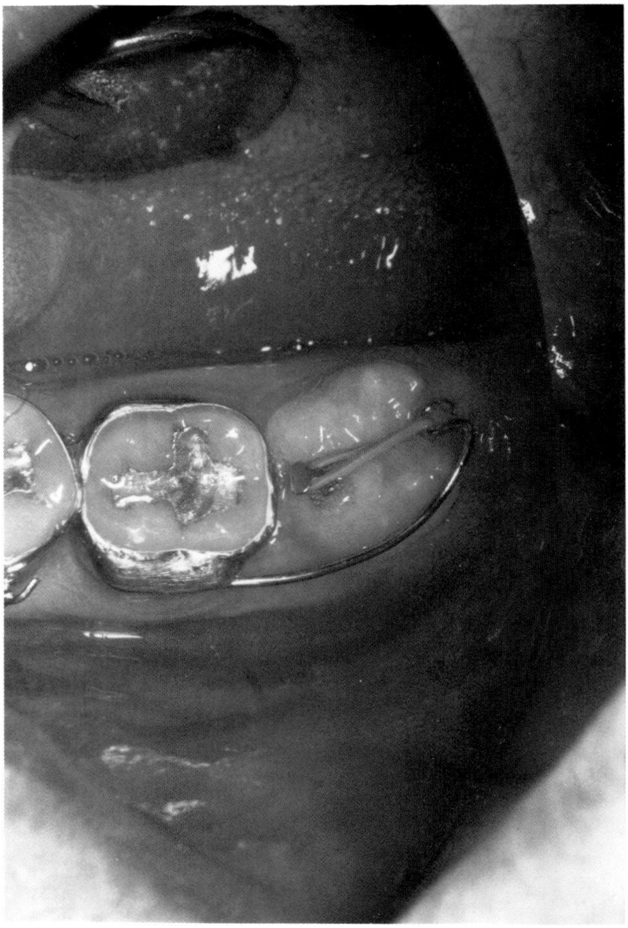

Figure 19. Third molar uprighting appliance in position after surgical exposure and healing (occlusal view).

sistent across eruption status, with a bias toward predicting eruption (importantly, this is contrary to most other prediction schemes, which are biased toward extraction). This test points out several aspects of the current status of prediction analysis involving third molars. Using a rather extensive list of possible variables, including those measures presently used in various prediction schemes, prediction efficiency, tested appropriately on another sample, did not produce an accuracy level consistent with that currently claimed. Nor were all of the variables used in other prediction schemes selected by the discriminant function analysis in this test. Such occurrences should cast further doubt on the value and accuracy of current prediction schemes. Further work is necessary; for now, it is sufficient to note that it appears that both anatomic and dental factors predispose to eruption or impaction of the third molars, and they are different for males and females at different ages.

Third Molar Orthodontics. While available dental arch space is indeed an appropriate concern for most adolescent patients, additional arch space continues to become available through time. This might permit not only natural eruption of a third molar, but also the positioning of the third molar by orthodontic means (Slodov *et al.,* 1989). In fact, by adopting a bias that adults continue to grow and, thus, to gain arch space, and by considering an impacted third molar to be just another malposed tooth, this possibility becomes an immediate reality. A simple technique which is most effective in treating impacted third molars that are exposed or unexposed has been developed (Fig. 19). When used with conventional fixed appliances, this technique presents a viable option to extraction, surgical repositioning, or optimistically predicting eruption. It makes many of the surgical and pathological justifications for extraction academic. Figure 20 illustrates that, with proper intervention, this technique is simple and effective in positioning malposed third molars.

This manipulation is a perfect example of a direct application of knowledge of continuing growth and development in the adult; non-traditional concepts are being used to form the rationale for non-traditional treatment. The technique has already been demonstrated to be beneficial to patients. Such a technique will likely find greater utilization in the future; since non-extraction therapy is being recommended more frequently than in the past and, since increasing numbers of second molar extractions are being performed, clinicians will be faced with increasing numbers of malposed third molars, where the only good, responsible alternative is to bring the third molars into place.

CONCLUDING REMARKS

The ability to control growth and predict the outcome of orthodontic treatment is founded in a thorough understanding of the biological processes involved, and a complete knowledge of maturational events. Craniofacial biologists and clinicians have traditionally centered their research attention on periods of life where relatively rapid and obvious

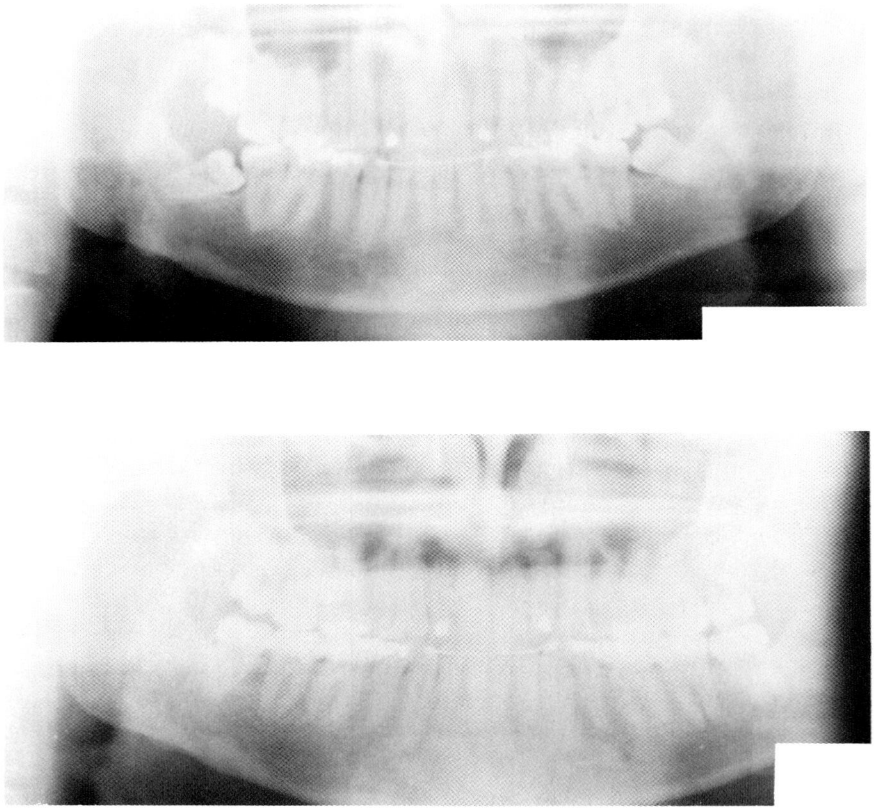

Figure 20. *Top.* Previously treated 18-year-old male patient with severe horizontal impactions of the lower third molars. *Bottom.* After molar uprighting and incorporation into regular fixed appliance therapy. Molar uprighting was accomplished in five months.

change is occurring. Typically, emphasis is given to the prenatal and early postnatal periods of life, up through adolescence. This has been productive, because the information is useful conceptually as a foundation for diagnosis and treatment planning, and clinically in development of methods for use in treatment. As the result of several decades of serious investigation, it is assumed that the growth of the craniofacial complex is a four-dimensional biological process that ends in the late teens or early twenties. In adulthood, the plasticity of bone is discounted, and the craniofacial complex is assumed to be static, stable, and final in form.

This restrictive "conventional wisdom" pervades the current orthodontic literature. However, in many other biological disciplines and through the efforts of recent research on the adult craniofacial skeleton, it is well substantiated that developmental mechanisms remain intact and changes in morphology continue throughout adulthood.

The consequences of adult growth are important clinically in several situations. While it is not likely that small increments of yearly growth will produce a ponderable impact on how we treat adult patients, knowledge of the amount and character of the change will impact decisions regarding diagnosis, relapse, and retention, when considering the eruption or extraction of third molars, when using maturity indicators for the purpose of timing both orthodontic and orthognathic treatments, and will in small but important ways impact the treatment of adolescents.

More important is accepting the concept that adults change, teeth move, and growth continues in spite of short-term attempts at alteration. By doing so, practitioners are apt to be less frustrated and better able to understand their patients, and their treatments may be better predicted and controlled.

REFERENCES

Andrew, R. *The Anatomy of Aging in Man and Animals.* Grune and Stratton, New York, 1971.

Bandeen, R.L. and T.A. Timm. Temporomandibular joint dysfunction: Report of a case. Am. J. Orthod. *87:*275-279, 1985.

Barrow, G.V. and J.R. White. Developmental changes of the maxillary and mandibular dental arches. Angle Orthod. *22:*41-46, 1952.

Behrents, R.G. A treatise on the continuum of growth in the aging craniofacial skeleton. Doctoral dissertation, The University of Michigan, Ann Arbor, 1984.

Behrents, R.G. *Growth in the Aging Craniofacial Skeleton.* Monograph 17, Craniofacial Growth Series, The Center for Human Growth and Development, The University of Michigan, Ann Arbor, 1985*a*.

Behrents, R.G. *An Atlas of Growth in the Aging Craniofacial Skeleton.* Monograph 18, Craniofacial Growth Series, Center for Human Growth and Development, The University of Michigan, Ann Arbor, 1985*b*.

Behrents, R.G. The biological basis for understanding craniofacial growth during adulthood. In: *Normal and Abnormal Bone Growth: Basic and Clinical Research.* A.D. Dixon and B.G. Sarnat (Eds.), Alan R. Liss, Inc., New York, 1985*c*.

Behrents, R.G and E.F. Harris. Timing orthognathic surgery according to adult growth. Proc. Am. Assoc. Orthod./Am. Assoc. Oral Maxillofac. Surg. Clin. Congr., 1986.

Behrents, R.G. and E.F. Harris. Normal length changes in hand bones during adulthood: Exploratory study of ray two. Ann. Hum. Biol. *14:*277-383, 1987.

Bibby, R.E. A cephalometric study of sexual dimorphism. Am. J. Orthod. *76:*256-259, 1979.

Bishara, S.E. and G.F. Andreason. Third molars: A review. Am. J. Orthod. *83:*131-137, 1983.

Bishara, S.E. and P.S. Burkey. Second molar extractions: A review. Am. J. Orthod. *89:*415-424, 1986.

Bishara, S.E. and J.R. Jakobsen. Longitudinal changes in three normal facial types. Am. J. Orthod. *88:*466-502, 1985.

Broadbent, B.H., Sr., B.H. Broadbent, Jr. and W.H. Golden. *Bolton Standards of Dentofacial Developmental Growth.* St. Louis: C.V. Mosby Company, 1975.

Buchi, E.C. Anderung der Korperform bein erwachsenen Menschen, eine Untersuchung nach der Individual Methode. Anthrop. Forschr., Wein, 1950.

Carmen, R.N. A study of mandibular anterior crowding in untreated cases and its interpretation. Master's thesis, Case Western Reserve University, Cleveland, 1978.

Chaconas, S.J. A statistical evaluation of nasal growth. Am. J. Orthod. *56:*403-414, 1969.

Chaconas, S.J. and J.D. Bartroff. Predication of normal soft tissue facial changes. Angle Orthod. *45:*12-25, 1975.

Christie, T.E. Cephalometric patterns of adults with normal occlusion. Angle Orthod. *47:*128-135, 1977.

Cleven, D. A longitudinal roentgenographic cephalometric investigation of mandibular growth in height, width and depth in males from early childhood to adulthood. Master's thesis, Northwestern University, Chicago, 1969.

Edwards, J.G. A study of the periodontium during orthodontic rotation of teeth. Am. J. Orthod. *54:*441-449, 1968.

Enlow, D.H. Personal communication, 1981.

Enlow, D.H. *Handbook of Facial Growth.* W.B. Saunders, Philadelphia, 1982.

Enlow, D.H., H.J. Bianco and S. Eklund. The remodeling of the edentulous mandible. J. Prosth. Dent. *36:*685-693, 1976.

Epker, B.N. and H.M. Frost. A histological study of remodeling at the periosteal, haversian canal, cortical endosteal and trabecular endosteal surfaces in human ribs. Anat. Rec. *152:*129-136, 1965.

Epker, B.N., M. Kelin and H.M. Frost. Magnitude and location of cortical bone loss in human rib with aging. Clin. Orthop. *41:*198-203, 1965.

Ericksen, M.F. Some aspects of aging in the lumbar spine. Am. J. Phys. Anthrop. *45:*575-580, 1976.

Ericksen, M.F. Aging in the lumbar spine in L1 and L2. Am. J. Phys. Anthrop. *48:*241-246, 1978.

Finch, C.E and L. Hayflick. *Handbook of the Biology of Aging.* Van Nostrand Reinhold, New York, 1977.

Fink, R.D. Validation of contemporary techniques for the prediction of lower third molar impaction. Master's thesis, Case Western Reserve University, Cleveland, 1976.

Fishman, L.S. Radiographic evaluation of skeletal maturation. Angle Orthod. *52:*88-112, 1982.

Fishman, L.S. Maturational patterns and prediction during adolescence. Angle Orthod. *57:*178-193, 1987.

Forsberg, C.M. Growth changes in the adult face. Master's thesis, Karolinska Institutet, Stockholm, 1976.

Forsberg, C.M. Facial morphology and aging: A longitudinal investigation of young adults. Eur. J. Orthod. *1:*15-23, 1979.

Gallerano, R.L. Mandibular anterior crowding, a post-retention study. Master's thesis, University of Washington, Seattle, 1976.

Garn, S.M. *The Earlier Gain and the Later Loss of Cortical Bone.* Charles C Thomas, Springfield, 1970.

Garn, S.M. The course of bone gain and the phases of bone loss. Orthop. Clin. N. Am. *3:*503-520, 1972.

Garn, S.M. Contributions of the radiographic image to our knowledge of human growth. Am. J. Roent. *137:*231-239, 1981.

Garn, S.M., C.G. Rohman and B. Wagner. Bone loss as a general phenomenon in man. Fed. Proc. *26:*1729-1736, 1967.

Garn, S.M., B. Wagner, C.G. Rohman and W. Ascoli. Further evidence of continuing bone expansion. Am. J. Phys. Anthrop. *28:*219-222, 1968.

Garn, S.M., K.P. Hertzog, A.K. Poznansky and J.M. Nagy. Metacarpophalangeal length in the evaluation of skeletal malformations. Radiology *105:*375-381, 1972.

Gibson, J.E., Jr. Stability of LeFort I osteotomies on growing patients: A longitudinal study. Master's thesis, University of Tennessee, Memphis, 1987.

Goggans, G.G. Skeletal and dental characteristics of individuals with erupted or impacted third molars: A longitudinal study. Master's thesis, University of Tennessee, Memphis, 1986.

Goldsman, S. The variations in skeletal and denture patterns in excellent adult facial types. Angle Orthod. *29:*63-92, 1959.

Graber, T.M. Postmortems in post-treatment adjustment. Am. J. Orthod. *52:*331-352, 1966.

Gregerman, R.I. and E.L. Beirman. Aging and hormones. In: *Textbook of Endocrinology.* 5th Ed., R.H. Williams (Ed.), W.B. Saunders, Philadelphia, 1974.

Haas, A.J. Let's take a rational look at permanent second molar extraction. Am. J. Orthod. *90:*361-363, 1986.

Hägg, U. and J. Taranger. Skeletal changes of the hand wrist as indicators of the pubertal growth spurt. Acta Odont. Scand. *38:*187-200, 1980.

Hägg, U. and J. Taranger. Maturation indicators and the pubertal growth spurt. Am. J. Orthod. *82:*299-309, 1982.

Harris, E.F. and R.G. Behrents. The intrinsic stability of Class I molar relationship: A longitudinal study of untreated cases. Am. J. Orthod. 1988, in press.

Harrison, M.A. Class II malocclusions: A longitudinal study of cephalometric and hand-wrist radiographs. Master's thesis, University of Tennessee, Memphis, 1986.

Hellman, M. An introduction to the growth of the human face from infancy to adulthood. Int. J. Orthod. *18:*777-798, 1932.

Hellman, M. The face in its developmental career. Dent. Cosmos *77:*685-787, 1935.

Hellman, M. Our third molar teeth, their eruption, presence, and absence. Dent. Cosmos *78:*750-762, 1936.

Hellman, M. Some aspects of wisdom teeth and their impaction. Arch. Clin. Oral Path. *2:*125-141, 1938.

Hellman, M. Development of the face and dentition in its application to orthodontic treatment. Am. J. Orthod. *26:*424-447, 1940.

Hixon, E. and P. Klein. Simplified mechanics: A means of treatment based on available scientific information. Am. J. Orthod. *62:*113-141, 1972.

Hotz, R. Paradontale Reaction auf Starke Krafte bei Dehandlung mit festsitzenden Apparaten. Fortschr. Kieferorthop. *27:*2, 1966.

Hunter, C.J. The correlations of facial growth with body height and skeletal maturation at adolescence. Angle Orthod. *36:*44-54, 1966.

Hunter, W.S. and S.M. Garn. Disproportionate sexual dimorphism in the human face. Am. J. Phys. Anthrop. *36:*133-138, 1981.

Ingerslev, C.H. and B. Solow. Sex differences in craniofacial morphology. Acta Odontol. Scand. *33:*85-94, 1975.

Israel, H. Loss of bone and remodeling—Redistribution in the craniofacial skeleton with age. Fed. Proc. *26:*1723-1728, 1967.

Israel, H. Continuing growth in the human cranial skeleton. Arch. Oral Biol. *13:*133-137, 1968.

Israel, H. The impact of aging upon the adult craniofacial skeleton. Master's thesis, University of Alabama, Birmingham, 1971.

Israel, H. Progressive enlargement of the vertebral body as part of the process of human skeletal aging. Age and Aging *2:*71-79, 1973.

Israel, H. The dichotomous pattern of craniofacial expansion during aging. Am. J. Phys. Anthrop. *47:*47-52, 1977.

Johnson, J.V. and G.P. Quirk. Surgical repositioning of impacted mandibular second molar teeth. Am. J. Orthod. *91:*242-251, 1987.

Johnston, L.E., Jr. A comparative analysis of Class II treatments. In: *Science and Clinical Judgment in Orthodontics.* P.S. Vig and K.A. Ribbens (Eds.), Monograph 19, Craniofacial Growth Series, Center for Human Growth and Development, The University of Michigan, Ann Arbor, 1986.

Kapley, K. A study of factors relating to mandibular anterior crowding in orthodontically untreated individuals. Master's thesis, Case Western Reserve University, Cleveland, 1982.

Kemp, D.H. Orthodontic stability: Contributions from growth and treatment. Master's thesis, University of Tennessee, Memphis, 1986.

Kendrick, G.S. and H.L. Risinger. Changes in the anteroposterior dimensions of the human male skull during the third and fourth decades of life. Anat. Rec. *159:*77-81, 1967.

Kincaid, J.J. Third molar eruption: Predictive methods. Master's thesis, University of Tennessee, Memphis, 1987.

Kohn, R.R. *Principles of Mammalian Aging.* Prentice-Hall, Englewood Cliffs, 1978.

Leydard, B.C. Study of the mandibular third molar area. Am. J. Orthod. *39:*366-372, 1953.

Little, R.M., R.T. Wallen and R.A. Riedel. Stability and relapse of mandibular anterior alignment—First premolar extraction cases treated by traditional edgewise orthodontics. Am. J. Orthod. *80:*349-365, 1981.

MacDowell, J.N. *MacDowell Orthodontia.* Blakely Printing Co., Chicago, 1901.

McNamara, J.A., Jr. Dentofacial adaptations in adults following functional regulator therapy. Am. J. Orthod. *85:*57-71, 1983.

Miller, S.C., J.G. Shupe, E.H. Redd, J.A. Miller and T.H. Omura. Changes in bone mineral and bone formation rates during pregnancy and lactation in rats. Bone *7:*283-287, 1986.

Moorrees, C.F.A. *The Dentition of the Growing Child. A Longitudinal Study of Dental Development Between 3 and 18 Years of Age.* Harvard University Press, Cambridge, 1959.

Muchnic, H.V. Retention or continuing treatment. Am. J. Orthod. *57:*23-34, 1970.

Nemeth, R.B. and R.J. Isaacson. Vertical anterior relapse. Am. J. Orthod. *65:*565-585, 1974.

Pool, G.L. The clinimetric impact of age and sex on orthodontic therapy. Master's thesis, University of Tennessee, Memphis, 1987.

Pfeiffer, S. Age changes in the external dimensions of adult bone. Am. J. Phys. Anthrop. *52:*529-532, 1980.

Reitan, K. Clinical and histological observations on tooth movement during and after orthodontic treatment. Am. J. Orthod. *53:*721-745, 1967.

Reitan, K. Principles of retention and avoidance of post-treatment relapse. Am. J. Orthod. *55:*776-790, 1969.

Ricketts, R.M. Studies leading to the practice of abortion of lower third molars. Dent. Clin. N. Am. *23:*393-410, 1979.

Ricketts, R.M., P.K. Turley, S. Chaconas and R.J. Schulhof. Third molar enucleation: Diagnosis and technique. J. Cal. Dent. Assoc. *4:*52-57, 1976.

Riolo, M.L., R.E. Moyers, J.A. McNamara, Jr. and W.S. Hunter. *An Atlas of Craniofacial Growth: Cephalometric Standards for the University School Growth Study.* Monograph 2, Craniofacial Growth Series, Center for Human Growth and Development, The University of Michigan, Ann Arbor, 1975.

Ruff, C.B. and W.C. Hayes. Subperiosteal expansion and cortical remodeling of the human femur and tibia with aging. Science *217:*945-947, 1982.

Sarnas, C.V. and B. Solow. Early adult changes in the skeletal and soft-tissue profile. Eur. J. Orthod. *2:*1-12, 1980.

Schudy, G.F. Post-treatment craniofacial growth: Its implications in orthodontic treatment. Am. J. Orthod. *65:*39-57, 1974.

Schulhof, R.J. Third molars and orthodonic diagnosis. J. Clin. Orthod. *106:*272-281, 1976.

Sedlin, E.D., A.R. Villanueva and H.M. Frost. Variations in cross-section areas of rib cortex and bone. J. Gerontol. *18:*9-13, 1963.

Sinclair, D. *Human Growth after Birth.* Oxford University Press, New York, 1978.

Slodov, I., R.G. Behrents and D.P. Dobrowski. Clinical experience with third molar orthodontics. 1989, in press.

Smith, R.W., Jr. Dietary and hormonal factors in bone loss. Fed. Proc. *26:*1737-1746, 1967.

Smith, R.W. and B. Frame. Concurrent axial and appendibular osteoporosis. New Engl. J. Med. *273:*73, 1967.

Smith, R.W. and R.R. Walker. Femoral expansion in aging women: Implications for osteoporosis and fractures. Science *145:*156-157, 1964.

Solow, B. The dentoalveolar compensatory mechanism: Background and clinical implications. Br. J. Orthod. *7:*145-161, 1980.

Susanne, C. Individual age changes of the morphological characteristics. J. Hum. Evol. *6:*181-189, 1977.

Subtelny, J.D. A longitudinal study of soft tissue facial structures and their profile characteristics, defined in relation to the underlying skeletal structures. Am. J. Orthod. *45:*481-507, 1959.

Tallgren, A. Neurocranical morphology and aging: A longitudinal roentgen cephalometric study of adult Finnish women. Am. J. Phys. Anthrop. *41:*285, 1974.

Thompson, J.L. and G.S. Kendrick. Changes in the vertical dimensions of the human male skull during the third and fourth decades of life. Anat. Rec. *150:*209-214, 1964.

Trotter, M., G.E. Broman and R.R. Peterson. Densities of bones of white and negro skeletons. J. Bone Joint Surg. *42A:*50-58, 1960.

Tulloch, J.F.C. and A.A. Antczak-Bouckoms. Decision analysis in the evaluation of clinical strategies for the management of mandibular third molars. J. Dent. Ed. *51:*652-660, 1987.

Turley, P.K. and S.J. Chaconas. A computerized method of forecasting third molar space in the mandibular arch. A.A.D.R Abstract, *54:*46-55, 1975.

Vanarsdall, R.L. and D.R. Musich. Adult orthodontics: Diagnosis and treatment. In: *Orthodontics: Current Principles and Techniques.* T.M. Graber and B.F. Swain (Eds.). C.V. Mosby Co., St. Louis, 1985.

Wei, S.H.Y. Craniofacial variations, sex differences, and the nature of prognathism in Chinese subjects. Angle Orthod. *39:*303-315, 1969.

Williams, R.A. Cranial and dental factors affecting long-term stability of the dental arch. Master's thesis, University of Tennessee, Memphis, 1985.

Williams, R.E. The influence of jaw growth on molar position, overjet, and mandibular plane angle. Master's thesis, University of Oregon, Eugene, 1971.

"GROWTH" AND AGING IN THE ADULT CRANIOFACIAL SKELETON

Donald H. Enlow

The term "aging" carries many common connotations. Some of these relate to somatic and physiologic changes that have been observed to precede a variety of degenerative body conditions; e.g., dementia, heart problems, vascular insufficiencies, arthritis, diabetes, declining lung capacity, tissue atrophy and cell death, sensory failures, immune system deficiencies, compromises in certain other vital functions, muscle weakening, loss of brain cells, decreased coordination, prostatic problems, compression of the spine, and so on. Researchers investigating the biologic conditions that underlie the aging process seem now to have settled into two groups. One advocates "wear and tear" theories, and the other espouses intrinsic "time-clock" concepts. For the former, the idea is that body functions sooner or later begin to yield to years of functional stress, or to cumulative DNA mutations, losses of key genes, activation of latent but detrimental genes, long-term accumulations of cellular glucose and lipofuscin, or the build-up of unstable free radicals. The clock theorists, on the other hand, hold that a built-in, pre-programmed genetic timer establishes a prescribed post-maturational period for the onset of cell death, perhaps by activation of some kind of killer hormone that begins to accumulate after sexual maturity, or, perhaps, by some pre-set genetic limit to a cell's life and ability to metabolize.

All changes related to aging, however, are not debilitating; some function advantageously in necessary responses to a variety of changing internal and environmental conditions. Many researchers acknowledge that, whatever the nature of the many constructive or destructive aging changes, *development* is a component part of the process. This is a conceptual point that bears on the present discussion regarding continuing craniofacial changes beyond childhood.

Cold-blooded (poikilothermic) vertebrates grow either continuously or seasonally as long as they live, becoming ever larger in whole body size. Conversely, among mammals, which are homeothermic, closure of the epiphyses around the time of reproductive maturity precludes continuing linear skeletal and body increases, with definitive adult stature established at this stage. Morphogenesis of all organ systems has become complete, and "growth" is perceived to essentially have ceased.

"Growth?" In the adult? That word seems misplaced. Something else must be going on. But then, after all, hair and fingernails continue to grow. Body weight usually increases during middle age. Dermal and mucosal epithelia are replaced throughout life. Teeth continue to drift and erupt. But are not those fundamental changes in adult craniofacial structure, as outlined by Dr. Behrents in this volume, really in some different category from such ordinary cell or tissue replacements or fluctuations? Further, should those facial changes not more appropriately be put under some special heading to distinguish them in principle from the childhood kind of growth, which seems essentially different?

With Dr. Behrents' revelations, where are we? The term "growth," as traditionally used by scholars and lay persons alike, has multiple connotations. For morphologists and clinicians, the term can mean almost anything a user intends it to mean, at whatever level of biologic sophistication. For example, the condyle is a principal "growth site." The face "grows" forward and downward (even though everyone is quite aware that the actual tissue growth activity is mostly upward and backward). It is frequently stated that some given orthodontic appliance stimulates or retards "growth," without specification of just what cellular or tissue changes might be involved. The point to be emphasized is that the word "growth," when applied to adult craniofacial changes, is quite acceptable *if* both the user of the word and the listener or reader understand the underlying biology.

An elementary but fundamental concept in facial morphogenesis is that there are two basic categories of *growth movement:* remodeling and displacement. The importance of awareness of this principle in practical clinical application cannot be overemphasized. Together, these two kinds of growth movements embody the expression of all the biologic activities converging to produce "growth." They are also the separate or combined targets of all orthodontic procedures, in the child and the adult alike.

"Remodeling" of hard or soft tissue involves five basic and essential phenomena: (1) size change; (2) establishment and progressive modifications of configuration; (3) relocations of parts (e.g., muscle migrations and shifts of parts into changed locations, as for the ramus or palate); (4) "fine-tuned" fitting of all separate parts to each other as they all continue to grow and change; and (5) continuous adjustments of all parts to multiple changes in intrinsic and extrinsic conditions.

Each of these aspects of the process of remodeling (which *is* "growth") is *also* involved in the adult kinds of changes described by Dr. Behrents. Significantly, many of these *same* aspects of the biologic process of remodeling that are associated with childhood growth continue throughout adulthood. Therefore, we can assert that *growth is an ongoing process of change that continuously seeks a state of structural and functional equilibrium, regardless of age.* Changes in environmental conditions, and the responses to these changes, are continuous and ceaseless throughout life. Muscles, for example, during and after childhood, undergo long-term changes in force potential, mass and action. Signals are emitted that activate sensory cell membrane receptors within osteogenic connective tissues, producing the complementary remodeling of the bones associated with the muscles. A feedback process proceeds toward a state of balance which, if ever achieved, is followed by a transient shutdown of the activating signals, until some new imbalance is introduced that reactivates the growth/remodeling process. This relentless remodeling component of growth is a continuum, and the same kinds of cellular activities operative during childhood growth, such as osteoblastic and osteoclastic responses, continue in the adult as well.

The frequent addition of "and development" after the word growth emphasizes the morphogenic principle that growth is a differential process in which the developmental activities involved proceed at different times, by different regional amounts, in different regional directions, and at different regional rates. Some observers may feel that, rather than simply "growth," a more descriptive phrase for adult changes would be proper, say "post-maturational differentiation." Some observers may wish to coin a wholly new word for a special category of growth. It is more likely, however, that most of us will simply continue to use the old words: growth, development, and remodeling, which are quite descriptive enough. What lie ahead now will be attempts to uncover in more depth the multiple conditions that underlie and predispose these adult changes, and to utilize this knowledge and develop methods for working with them for clinical advantage.

ORTHODONTIC TREATMENT OF THE DEGENERATED DENTITION

Birte Melsen

Not many years ago, it was normal for elderly people to lose all their natural teeth. Degeneration of the dentition was the first step along the inevitable road toward a full denture. It is thus not surprising that many artists, when portraying older people, made it obvious that their subjects had no remaining natural teeth (Fig. 1). Indeed, images of elderly persons that show a profile view often reveal other characteristics in addition to dental status, e.g., loss of vertical facial height and prognathism of the lower jaw, that are characteristic of edentulous individuals. These features reflect a negative stereotypic view of aging, i.e. that an older person is without power, without sexual attractiveness, and heading toward the end of life. In some depictions, edentulous elderly persons are made to look slightly ridiculous, and even pathetic (Fig. 2).

Teeth are more than just a component of the chewing apparatus. Psychologically, teeth seem to have a much deeper meaning. For example, Jung (1982, 1984) indicated in his dream analysis that dreaming about loss of teeth is highly related to the fear of losing power—professionally, economically, or sexually. According to Freud (1983), dreams about dental care are related to masturbation. More generally, extraction of permanent teeth due to decay has been related to fear of death, and has been perceived as the first sign of a general physical degeneration (Freud, 1983). Maintenance of natural teeth, therefore, has implications that extend far beyond sustaining optimal chewing function. Preserving the natural dentition can greatly influence the quality of life and a person's self perception (Melsen *et al.*, 1987*a*).

The relationships between the condition of the dentition and the well-being of the individual were noted by Goldstein, who stated that "protruding teeth [and] spacing of teeth...are frequent causes of much unhappiness for many people" (1968). Seide commented that "certainly nothing will make a person feel older than losing some or all of the teeth" (1976). Many adults seek orthodontic or prosthodontic care as a therapy for deeply rooted emotional problems.

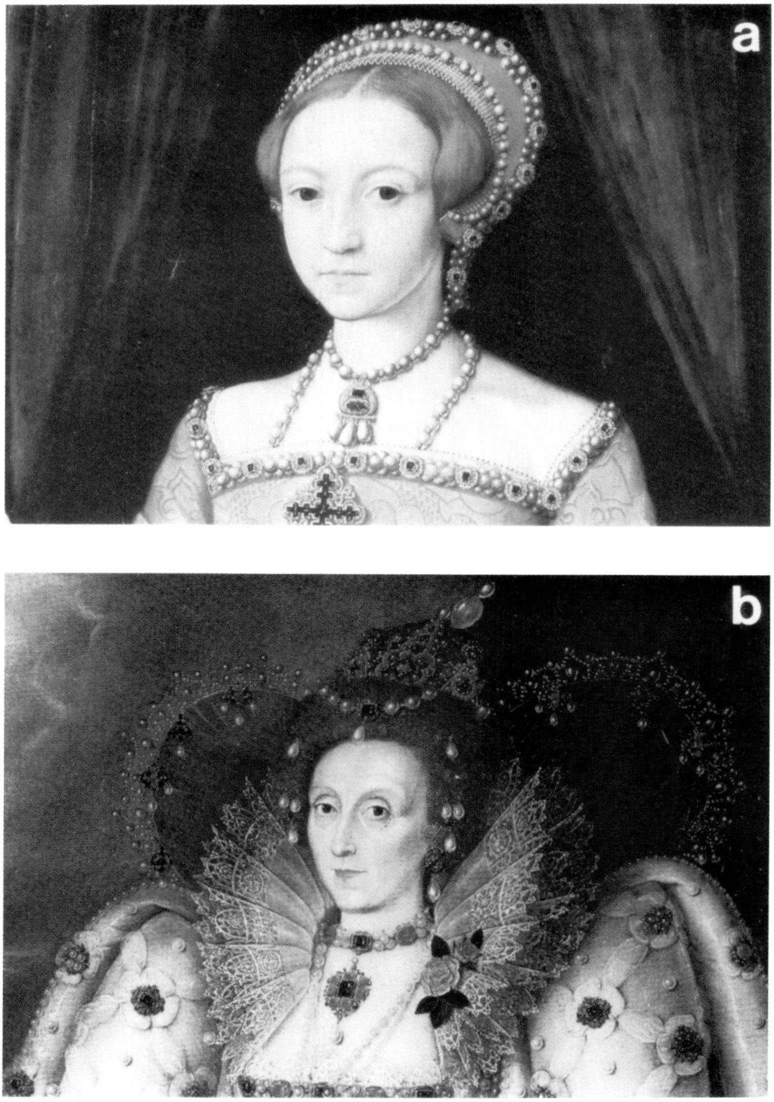

Figure 1. Two portraits of Elizabeth I of England. *A*. Elizabeth I as Princess (Anonymous, Royal Collection, London; used with permission). *B*. Loss of alveolar prognathism and temporal muscle mass, both of which are characteristics of the edentulous person, are evident. (Marcus Gheeraerts: *The Younger Elizabeth the First*, 1592. By courtesy of the National Portrait Gallery, London.)

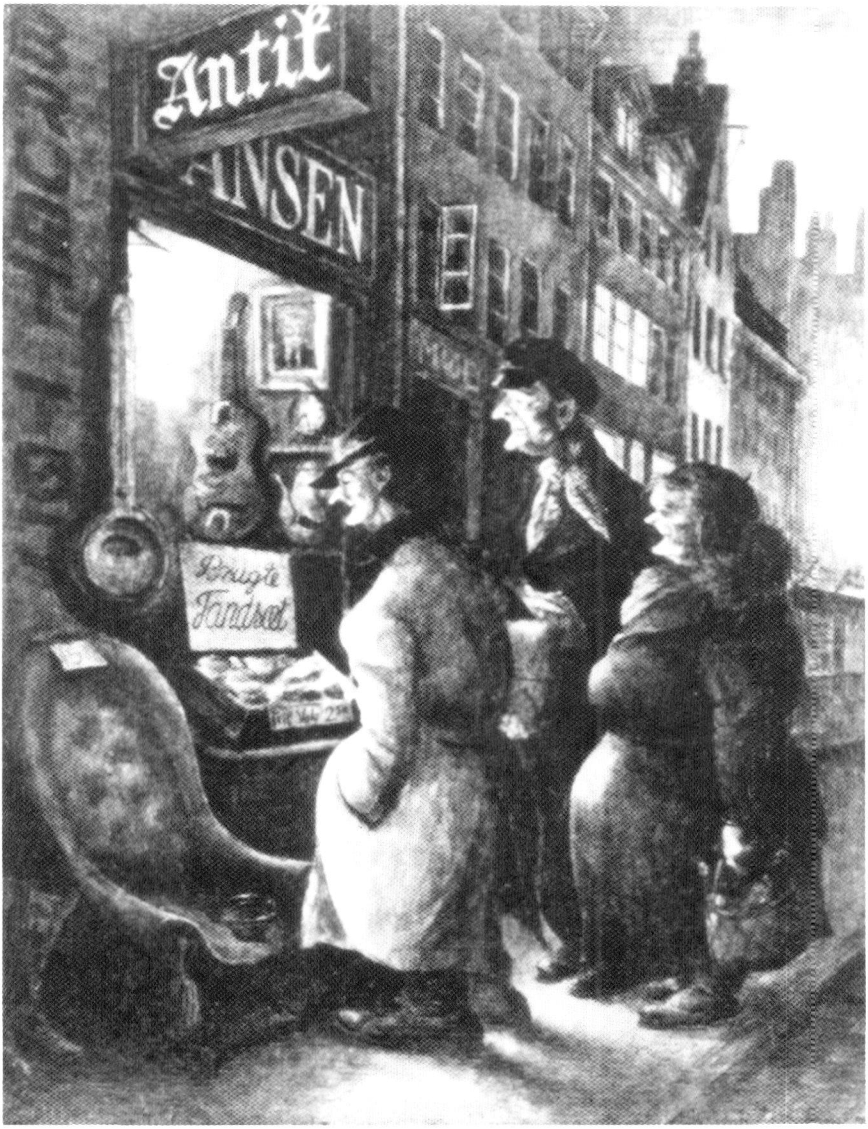

Figure 2. Drawing by Harald Engman of older people looking for used dentures in which the characteristics of the edentulous are made grotesque and ridiculous. (By courtesy of Munksgaard, Copenhagen.)

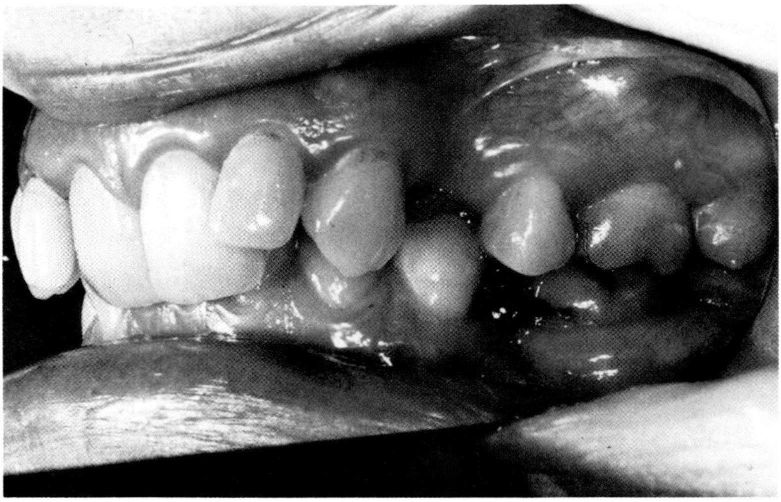

Figure 3. Example of a malocclusion that developed following extraction of four first premolars. In the lower jaw, the extraction space was closed through lingual tipping of the incisor segment. In the upper jaw, the incisors are crowded in spite of the extraction. A deepening of the bite, with gingival impingement, resulted from the extraction.

The influence of a degenerating dentition on an individual's life is also related to their ethnic and cultural background as well as their educational and socio-economical level (Melsen *et al.,* 1987*a*). For certain groups in Africa and Australia, the loss or mutilation of selected teeth are considered symbols of dignity or maturity (van Reenen, 1978; Briedenhann and van Reenen, 1985; van Reenen and Briedenhann, 1986). In cultures where age is related to experience and wisdom and assigned an important role in the society, age-related changes in appearance are not perceived as undesirable, but as signs of dignity and wisdom. In the Western world today, on the other hand, youth and fitness are considered desirable and high priority is given to the maintenance of a youthful appearance through body maintenance, fashion and cosmetics. In this context, teeth are important. It has gradually become less acceptable to have natural teeth replaced by dentures.

This paper deals with the treatment aspects of the degenerating dentition. The focus will be on the general principles of treatment planning and selection of biomechanics for the adult patient presenting a degenerating dentition. Special attention will be paid to the treatment of elongated spaced incisors developed as a result of advanced periodontal disease, and to the re-establishment of valid posterior segments where previous extraction has been followed by tipping and/or rotation of molars and atrophia of the alveolar process. It will be demonstrated how tooth movement with, and not through, bone can help rebuild the alveolar processes and improve the attachment level. Five selected cases will be presented as examples of the complexity of orthodontic treatment in this type of patient.

DEGENERATION OF THE DENTITION

The etiology of the degeneration of the dentition is usually related to one or more of the following factors: (1) loss of teeth, (2) loss of periodontal support, and (3) decrease in general bone density.

Loss of Teeth

In the extraction of even a single tooth, the equilibrium of the dentition is interrupted and a spontaneous migration, often expressed as tipping and rotation of the adjacent teeth, can take place. Overeruption of teeth lacking occlusal contact can also occur. In the lower jaw, the extraction space will often close partly from the anterior aspect, thus leading to an increase in overbite (Fig. 3) and overjet. If the balance of the incisor contact is disturbed, a continued deterioration may take place, resulting in further anterior displacement of the upper incisors; once the lower lip is being caught by the upper incisors, they will be displaced forwardly more rapidly.

Loss of Periodontal Support

With apical displacement of the marginal bone level, the center of resistance is displaced in an apical direction. Burstone and Pryputniewicz (1980) found by means of laser holography that the center of resistance is normally localized 40% of the distance from the marginal bone level to the apex of an incisor tooth. Since incisors are subject to oblique and horizontal forces through biting and chewing, a moment tipping the teeth forward is generated. This moment is the state of equilibrium kept in balance by the external muscle matrix. With increasing distance from the point of contact to the center of resistance, the increased moment gen-

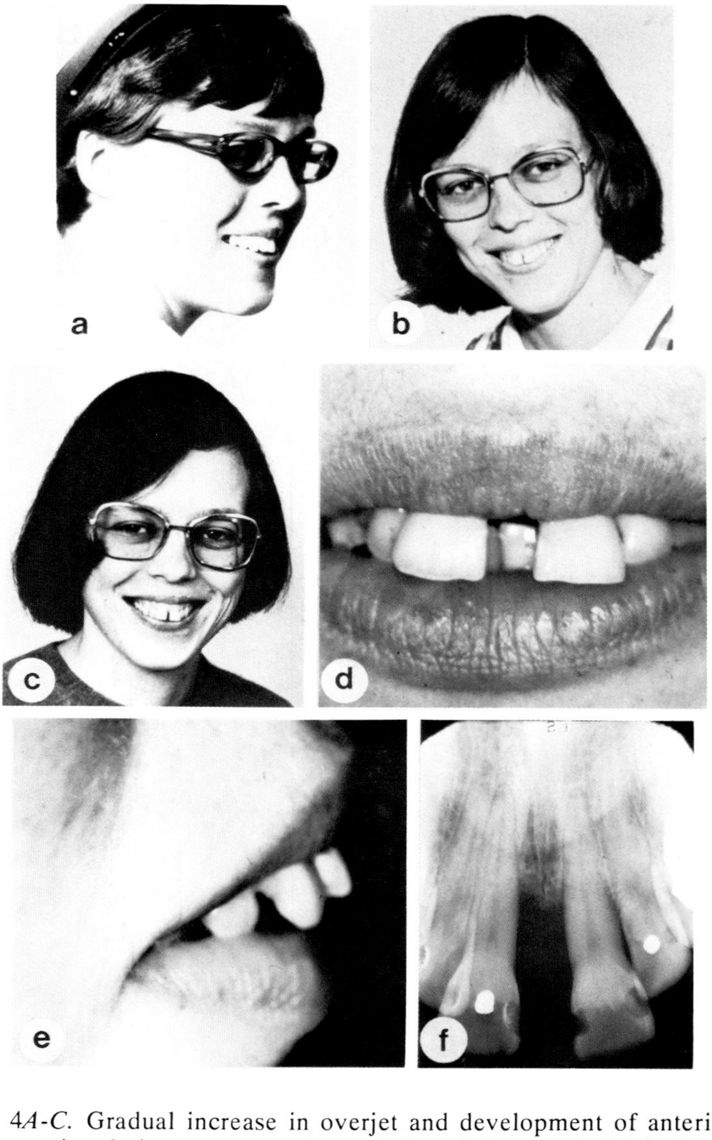

Figure 4*A-C*. Gradual increase in overjet and development of anterior diastema, seen in relation to progressing periodontal disease. *D,E*. Lip-incisor relationship before treatment. *F*. Periapical status of incisors before treatment.

erated leads to anterior tipping of the teeth. The same vicious cycle as described above may be the result (Fig. 4).

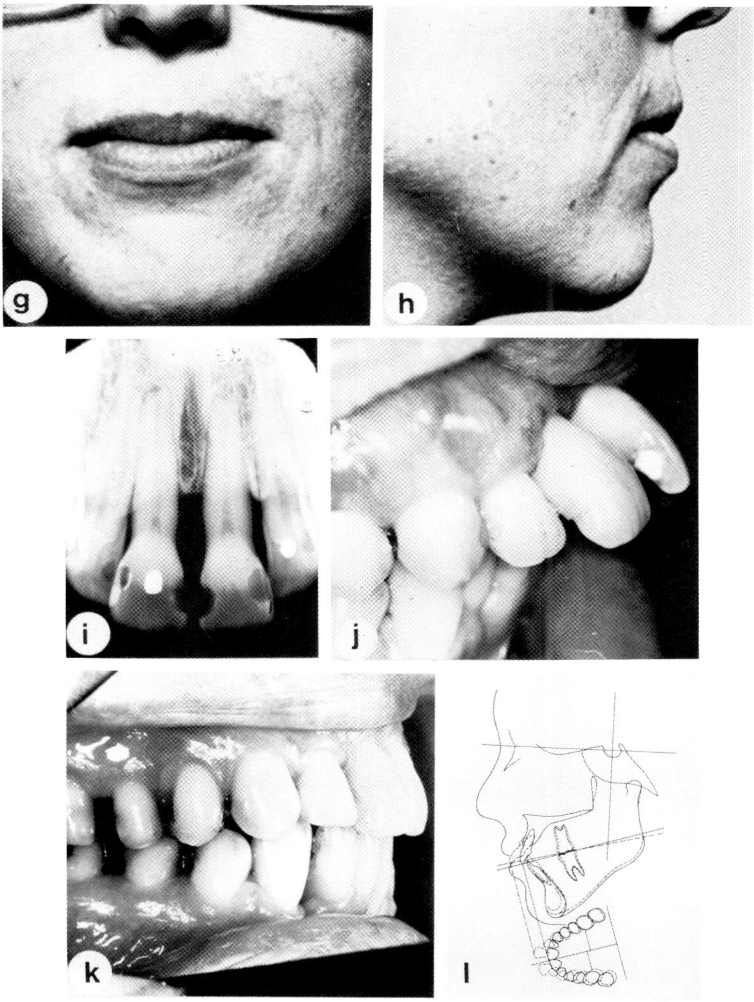

Figure 4, continued. *G, H.* Lip-incisor relationship after treatment. *I.* Periapical status after treatment. *J.* Occlusion before treatment. *K.* Occlusion after treatment. *L.* Treatment objective before treatment. Combination of profile radiograph and occlusogram offers the possibility of an establishment of the desired tooth movement in three dimensions, here illustrated in a case exhibiting an increased overjet, deep bite crowding in the lower and spacing in the upper jaw. The profile radiograph illustrates the planned displacement of the incisors and the corresponding occlusogram the tooth movement in the upper jaw following extraction of one premolar.

Age-Related Bone Loss

With increasing age, a decrease occurs in the amount of bone. Specifically, the volume of the trabecular bone expressed as the percentage of total bone and marrow which is occupied by bony trabeculi decreases, while cortical bone decreases in width and increases in porosity (Melsen, 1978). This general trend is also seen in the alveolar process and is further influenced by the local factors mentioned above. The contour of the alveolar process is totally dependent on the presence of teeth, and following dental extraction, the alveolar process suffers from severe atrophy. "Disuse" osteoporosis likewise develops around a tooth that is not in occlusal contact (Picton, 1969).

In summary, it can be demonstrated that a number of age related factors decrease the resistance of the tissue supporting the teeth, i.e., the alveolar bone. Taken together, these factors facilitate spontaneous dental migration, leading to degeneration of the natural dentition.

Patient's Decision Process

The decision for orthodontic treatment is an important part of the total treatment, particularly in the adult (Vanarsdall and Musich, 1985). Most patients have a rather vague understanding of the functional and cooperative requirements involved in orthodontic treatment; it is, therefore, of utmost importance that the patient is thoroughly informed before the decision to proceed with orthodontic treatment is made. Generally, more than one type of orthodontic treatment is possible for an individual. The different alternatives have to be weighed against each other (Fig. 5). The financial consequences, the cooperation, and the time aspect all have to be taken into consideration. Post-orthodontic treatment is likewise important. The patient should be informed about retention, to what degree reconstruction is needed, and whether fixed or removable retention is likely to be needed for a limited or an extended period.

It is at this stage, i.e., before treatment is initiated, that the patient's expectations must be made concordant with the possible treatment. Most treatments of degenerating dentitions are compromise treatments, since the number of teeth present and the quality of periodontal support are usually not adequate to produce an optimal treatment result. The compromise must be accepted by the patient and must be within reach of the orthodontist's capabilities. It is important to avoid a situation in which the maximum achievable result falls far from the patient's expectations.

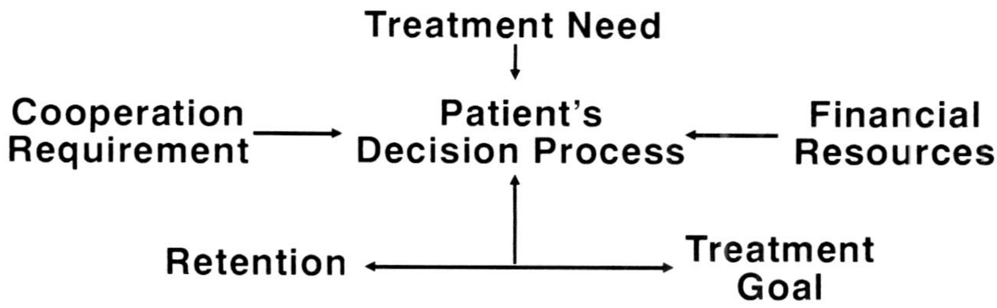

Figure 5. Factors influencing patient's decision regarding orthodontics.

INTERDISCIPLINARY COLLABORATION

During the decision process that is preliminary to orthodontic treatment of an adult patient, it is important for the orthodontist to communicate with colleagues (Musich, 1986*a,b*): the general practitioner, the family dentist, the periodontologist, and possibly the gnathologist may all be involved in the treatment simultaneously. It is very important that decay and endodontic problems are addressed before orthodontic treatment is initiated. In addition, orthodontic treatment should not be considered until the periodontium is in a healthy condition.

Thus, no detailed treatment plan should be agreed upon before the basic sequence of the total treatment is determined. Minor surgery such as local subapical osteotomies, which may occasionally be taken into consideration, require consultation with a surgeon, even if no orthognathic correction of the skeletal relationships is planned. Patients suffering from TMJ dysfunction should first be treated for these problems with splint therapy by a gnathologist or by an orthodontist as the first step of orthodontic treatment (see below).

During treatment, it is important that the patient's periodontal health is maintained. Although gingival inflammation in children does not always lead to periodontal disease, the host resistance is weakened in adults (Schei *et al.,* 1959; Lindhe, 1983) and orthodontic treatment of adults with periodontal disease will invariably lead to a deterioration of the tissues supporting the teeth.

ORTHODONTIC TREATMENT IN THE ADULT

Definition of Detailed Treatment Objectives

Once a decision is made regarding treatment, the necessary tooth movements must be determined in detail before a biomechanical system can be selected. In adult patients, only tooth movement and the subsequent modeling of the alveolar process can be performed orthodontically. Skeletal changes can only be produced through orthognathic surgery.

The first step in the orthodontic treatment procedure is to establish the mandibular position. This is particularly important for patients presenting symptoms from joints and/or muscles. In such patients, a mandibular position where the symptoms are relieved must be established; coincidence between intercuspation and the structural position, i.e., the position determined by joints and muscles, must be the treatment goal. This position will often be found through initial splint therapy as described by Møller (1981) and Møller and Bakke (1986). Once this position is achieved, it is maintained by a deep intercuspation produced in the splint. Tooth movement is then performed in areas where the splint has been reduced or removed.

In cases where no symptoms from chewing apparatus are present, the mandibular position as well as the cant of the occlusal plane must be maintained. As the stomatognathic system, i.e., the TMJ and the muscles of an adult patient, only rarely can tolerate increase in facial height, it is crucial to avoid extrusion of teeth in the side segments.

Following establishment of the mandibular position, the next step is to determine the desired tooth movement in three planes of space, giving the highest priority to the correction of the vertical discrepancies which, in most cases, include a deep bite. In the majority of adult patients, the deep bite should be solved through intrusion of incisor teeth without extrusion of molar teeth and the subsequent posterior rotation of the mandible (Melsen, 1986). Sagittal problems, large overjet, and spacing problems should usually be corrected through a combined retraction and intrusion of the incisors (Melsen, 1980). The treatment objective is simulated three-dimensionally through a combination of profile radiographs and occlusograms as previously described by Marcotte (1976) and later exemplified by Melsen (1986). (An example is seen in Figure 4).

Selection of Biomechanics

The selection of a biomechanical system depends on the amount and nature of the tooth displacement needed to reach the treatment objective (Burstone, 1985; Melsen, 1986). The segmented arch gives the option of differentiating clearly between the active appliance and the passive appliance (Burstone, 1982). For the active appliance, a configuration delivering the necessary moment-to-force ratio is selected. The choice of wire material and cross-section determines the force level and the load deflection rate. The passive appliance of the anchorage unit also requires special consideration in the degenerating dentition.

Vertical control during orthodontic treatment is a major issue, especially in adults since there is not sufficient growth to neutralize the undesirable effect of dental extrusion. Adequate vertical control can only be achieved if the segmented approach to biomechanics is utilized. In the segmented arch the dentition is treated as "two teeth," an entity that comprises an active and a reactive unit (Burstone and Koenig, 1974). While the teeth to be removed are in the active unit, the anchorage block is in the reactive unit. The segmented arch technique is a non-friction technique in which the teeth are moved by springs activated for the delivery of well-defined force systems (Burstone, 1962).

In adult patients, there is usually only a need for the displacement of a few teeth in relation to the remaining dentition, which thus serve as a reference.

Anchorage Preparation

The usual procedure of anchorage preparation, starting with leveling, cannot be applied to the adult patient. Through the so-called leveling, excessive forces including extrusive forces are produced (Burstone and Koenig, 1974, 1988; Ronay *et al.,* 1988), leading to loss of vertical control. The occlusion is also disturbed. Both of these factors preclude the possibility of utilizing the occlusion as part of the anchorage. The use of extraoral traction is rarely acceptable to elderly patients and further leads to an undesirable interaction with the force system used for orthodontic tooth movement (Thurow, 1975; Melsen, 1988).

Occlusal forces can be utilized as part of the anchorage and the impact of occlusion optimized if the occlusion is reinforced by means of a cemented splint. In this way, teeth which have no occluding contacts in the dentition can also be utilized. Reinforcement of the lateral anchorage units across the palate is also useful (Fig. 6*E*). Teeth that should remain mutually stable can be united by rigid wires bonded directly to the teeth, as is usually done with a retainer, or through the use of a splint to which the necessary tubes for the active appliance can be welded (Fig. 7*F*).

The Active Appliance

In relation to the active appliance, i.e., the appliance delivering the forces that produce tooth movement, it is important to realize that teeth can be moved either with bone or through bone (Fontenelle, 1986). Tooth movement with bone requires a balance between resorption and apposition during tooth movement, and can only be obtained in the absence of hyalinization and of local necroses of the periodontal ligament, which can result from excessive stress. Tooth movement must take place through direct resorption in one area and corresponding apposition in another area of the periodontal ligament; a controlled stress distribution is thus required. The absolute force magnitude is less important than the stress level, i.e., the force distribution or the force per unit of bone. These requirements are yet another reason for the use of the segmented arch system for tooth movement. Continuous arches simply do not allow for sufficient control of the force distribution, since it is determined entirely by the angle between wire and bracket in the single areas.

Correction of Special Elongated Incisors

A large number of the patients suffering from a degenerating dentition have incisors with excessive space and long clinical crowns. Until recently, it has been uncertain whether or not intrusion could be carried out and, if done, whether this tooth movement would not generate vertical defects and a deterioration of the periodontal status. However, recent clinical (Melsen *et al.,* 1988*a*) and experimental studies have demonstrated that the length of the clinical crown can be shortened through intrusion, without generation of a measurable pocket. Histological studies carried out on monkeys (Melsen *et al.,* 1988*b*) further verify that formation of a new attachment can be produced if the intruded teeth are surrounded by a reduced but healthy periodontium, in cases with horizontal bone loss but no vertical bone loss. An average of 1.49 mm of new attachment was observed following 12 to 16 weeks of intrusion of premolars which, at the start of treatment, were subject to a Widman flap operation with the purpose of removing the pocket epithelium and reducing the pocket depth. Regular curettage during intrusion was also part of the regime.

It seems important that the intrusion was performed with very light forces monitored to the existing periodontal support; 5 to 15 g per tooth has been found adequate to produce intrusion of single-rooted teeth.

The application of the above mentioned principles is illustrated in the following three case histories.

Case I (Fig. 6)

A 29-year-old pregnant woman was referred for preprosthetic orthodontics. The treatment plan included extraction and replacement with a bridge of one central incisor (21), which was severely periodontally involved. A lower molar which was lost earlier would likewise be replaced by a bridge. Since the incisal diastema did not permit construction of a bridge and the lower premolars were tilted distally into the extraction space, the reason for referral was to prepare the teeth for the planned restoration.

Clinical Examination. The permanent teeth were present except for 36 and 46, which had been extracted during childhood. 37 through 47 were mesially tipped; 34, 35 and 43 were distally tipped.

The Occlusion. The patient presented a distal molar relationship in the right side and a neutrocclusion on the left second molars. The canine relationship was a distocclusion on both sides. The overjet was 4 mm and the overbite 7 mm, with the central incisors the most elongated. There was marked spacing in the upper and lower incisor region. There was a non-occlusion in the right premolar region and a midline discrepancy of the lower mandible, 1.5 mm to the right. There was a general spacing in the incisor segment of both jaws.

Periodontal Status. Oral hygiene was satisfactory and the gingivae were healthy, but as a result of periodontal surgery, the clinical crowns were prolonged (Fig. 6*A, B*). There was a general bone loss of 50 to 80%, most pronounced in the incisor region of the maxilla. These incisors had third degree mobility (Ramfjörd, 1979). A functional analysis revealed marked bruxism facets on all upper incisors.

The cephalometric analysis clearly demonstrated an anteriorly rotated mandible and overerupted upper incisors.

Treatment Plan and Mechanics. It was determined that the maxillary side segments should be stabilized with lingually bonded 0.5 x 1.5 mm

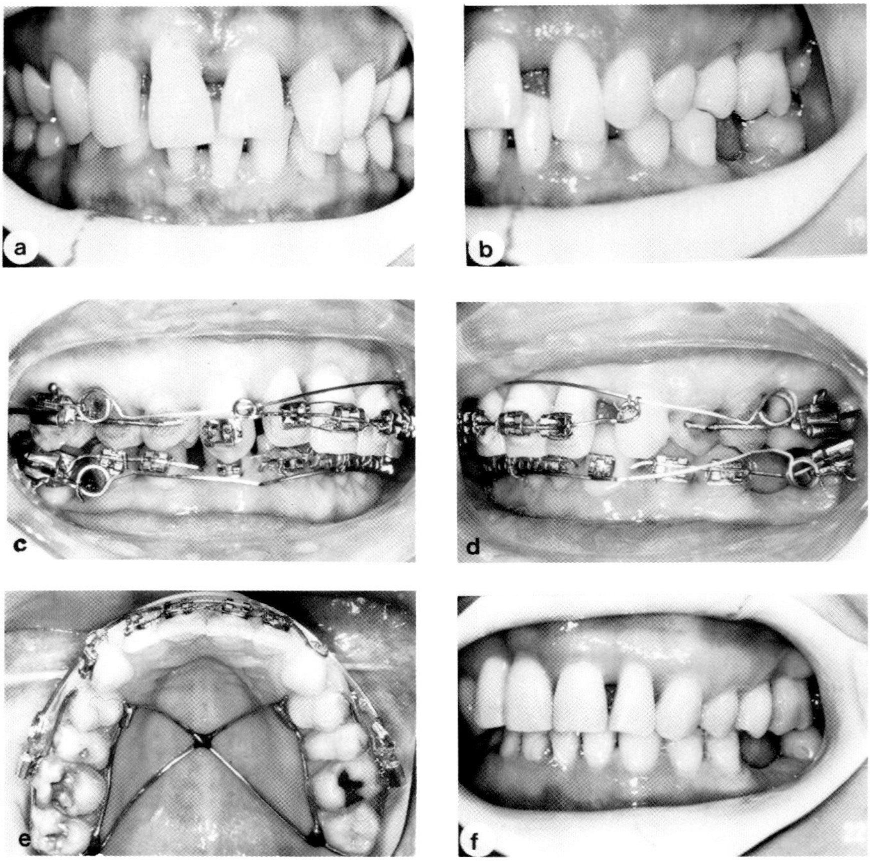

Figure 6. Case I. *A, B.* Pretreatment status. As a result of extrusive migration in relation to progressing periodontal disease, general diastemata and increased overbite developed. The periodontal surgery led to long clinical crowns but no pockets could be detected. *C, D.* The incisors were intruded by means of a base arch with a low force level (10 g per tooth). The anchorage consisted of a passive rigid wire system banded directly labially and lingually to the upper molar-premolar segment. *E.* The anchorage included two wires crossing the palate. *F.* Post-treatment status. Note the reduced clinical crown length. The gingival status was healthy.

wires, and 0.021 x 0.028 inch stainless steel wires to which wire pads had been welded, bonded labially. With this apparatus as anchorage, the upper incisors were intruded and slightly retracted by means of a base

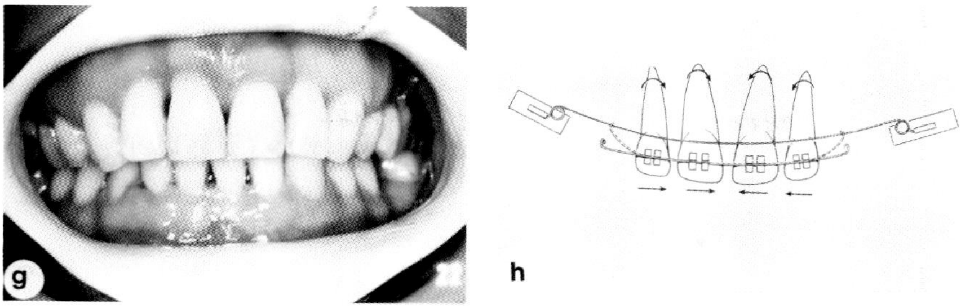

Figure 6, continued. *G.* Post-treatment status. *H.* Schematic drawing of intrusion mechanics.

arch generating 10 g intrusive force per tooth. Tooth number 21 was included in treatment for esthetic reasons, although its prognosis was dubious and it was planned for extraction. The most elongated teeth were treated by intrusion first.

In the lower jaw, the spacing of the incisors was to be reduced by slightly intruding and protruding them in order to develop a normal incisor relationship, and to tip 34 and 35 mesially, and 37 distally, and provide space for a bridge for replacement of 36. This decision was later altered since it seemed possible to develop a stable occlusion without reconstruction of the bridge.

Result. The treatment objective for the incisors was achieved: the clinical crown length was reduced and no pockets could be measured. Intraoral radiographs confirmed an improvement in the marginal bone level. Intercuspidation was in neutral occlusion on the left, and cusp to cusp on the right side. The periodontal condition had remained under control and incisor 21, which had been planned for extraction, was maintained. The result was retained by means of a splint worn 24 hours a day for three months and subsequently at night. It was not anticipated that the patient could maintain the treatment result without some sort of permanent retention. The upper incisors were therefore splinted by a twisted wire bonded to the lingual surface.

Case II (Fig. 7)

A 46-year-old male was referred for orthodontic treatment by a periodontologist. He was suffering from 70 to 80% marginal bone loss, but following a flap operation, no pockets above 3 mm were present. The upper left first premolar and the mesial root of the upper left first molar were lost due to periodontal deterioration. The patient was suffering from frequent headaches and had pain at palpation of the temporal and the medial pterygoid musculature. All teeth had second degree mobility, except for the incisors, which were loosened to the third degree. The occlusion was one premolar width distal and characterized by an extreme overjet and a deep bite, with impingement of the labial gingiva of the lower incisors. In the right side there was non-occlusion of the first premolar. Chewing ability was minimal, due to both the non-occlusion which prevented lateral movements, and the extreme loosening.

Treatment Objective. Since for this patient there was everything to gain and nothing to lose, an attempt was made to maintain all available teeth, and to re-establish a normal function and a normal overbite by means of intrusion of the incisor segment, with some bite opening to a degree that was tolerable for the patient. There was an obvious need for reconstruction work to stabilize the orthodontic result following treatment.

Treatment Sequence. In order to relieve the patient's muscle symptoms, an attempt was made to establish an occlusion on a cemented splint which was connected across the palate with 1.5 mm stainless steel wire welded to the splint on both sides (Fig. 7*F*). In this splint triple tubes were embedded buccally in the molar region. From the tubes a base arch of 0.18 inch TMA was constructed to give intrusion forces of 30-40 g on the four incisors. The force was added to "the anterior tooth unit" i.e., 0.018 x 0.025 inch stainless steel wire connecting the four incisors first with a rectangular loop wire in order to level the incisors segment and later with a heavy stainless steel 0.021 x 0.026 inch wire passively holding the four incisors together. In the lower jaw, two passive rigid side segments were established and the four incisors intruded by means of a base arch; following intrusion of the incisors, the canines were tilted slightly labially, and were also intruded.

After leveling and some intrusion of the upper incisors were achieved, the appliance was moved to the lingual side of the incisor (Fig. 7*F*). A wire to which a net base had been welded was bonded to the lingual side of the incisors, and the intrusion was continued lateral to the lateral incisors (where the base arch was tied to two small tubes welded to the wire connecting the incisors). Part of the splint was removed at that point, so that intrasplint tooth movement was possible.

Post-treatment Status. An adequately functioning dentition was re-established. The severe marginal bone loss necessitated permanent retention which was addressed, in part, through reconstruction in the molar

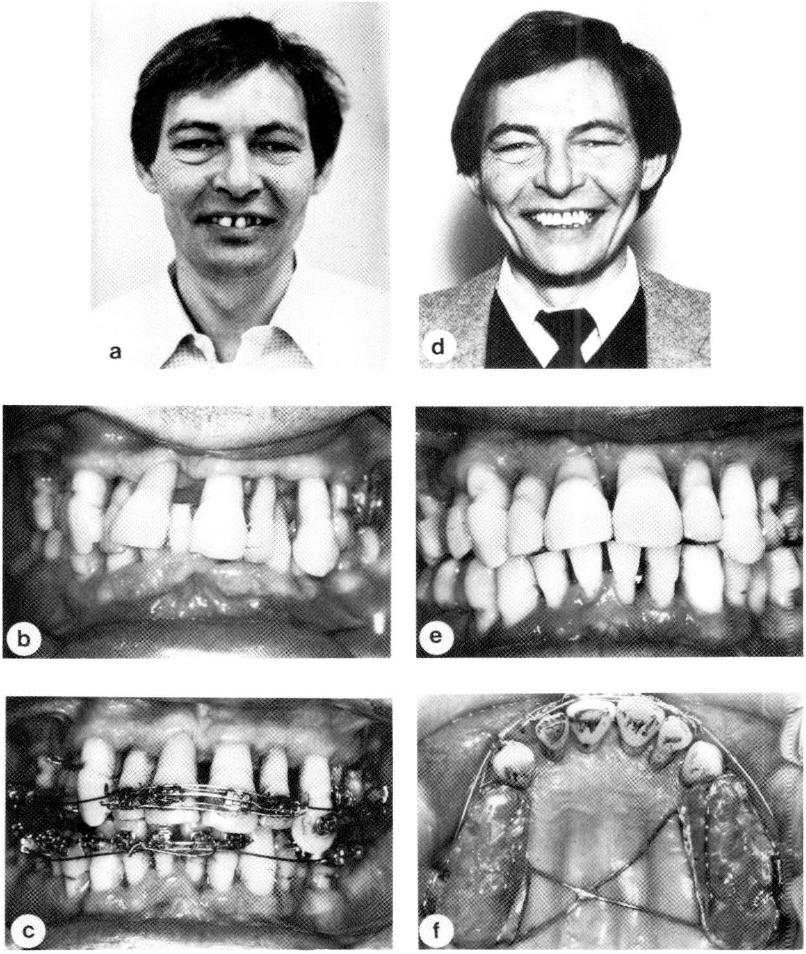

Figure 7. Case II. *A.* Pretreatment, extraoral view. *B.* Clinical status before treatment. *C.* Appliance used for intrusion and space closure. The incisors were intruded by means of a base arch with a low force level (5 to 10 g per tooth). *D, E.* Post-treatment status. Note the reduced clinical crown length. The gingival status was healthy. *F.* The anchorage included two wires crossing the palate.

region, where one root was missing. A bonded canine-to-canine retainer was inserted in both the upper and the lower jaw. The patient has benefited immensely by the treatment, physically as well as psychologically. The post-treatment observation period is three years and the patient seems to be able to maintain the result.

Case III (Fig. 8)

A 35-year-old woman had experienced extraction of all four first molars as a consequence of juvenile periodontitis. Following the extractions, the second molars were tilted into the extraction spaces. As a consequence of the reduced periodontium, spontaneous migration had taken place, especially in the incisor region. The upper right central incisor had third degree mobility (Ramfjörd, 1960), and was caught by the lower lip in speaking and swallowing. The other incisor had third degree mobility. This mobility caused great concern for the patient, particularly during chewing.

Pretreatment intraoral status showed that the incisors had lost 60 to 70% of the marginal bone. No marginal lamina dura was present in the molar region, probably due to lack of function.

Treatment. The patient was treated with a segmented arch wire appliance to produce intruding, retracting, and rotating of the protruded incisors.

Result. The post-treatment status showed that normal lip closure was re-established, and the clinical crowns were shortened. The incisor segment was retained by a bonded canine-to-canine retainer. The cross bite in the molar region had to be maintained, since this area was part of the passive rigid anchorage unit. One incisor in the lower jaw was extracted due to the advanced periodontitis.

X-rays taken after completion of treatment revealed that the bony support was improved, and in the molar region where no tooth movement had taken place, the density of the bone was increased due to improved function. Slight root resorption of the incisor had occurred, but as a whole, the periodontal support was improved. The treatment result has been stable for several years and the progression of the periodontal disease has been stopped.

Re-establishment of Valid Posterior Occlusion

Another category of patients requires orthodontic treatment as a preparation for reconstructional bridgework. Two different problems are frequently encountered: (1) mesially tilted second or third molars, and

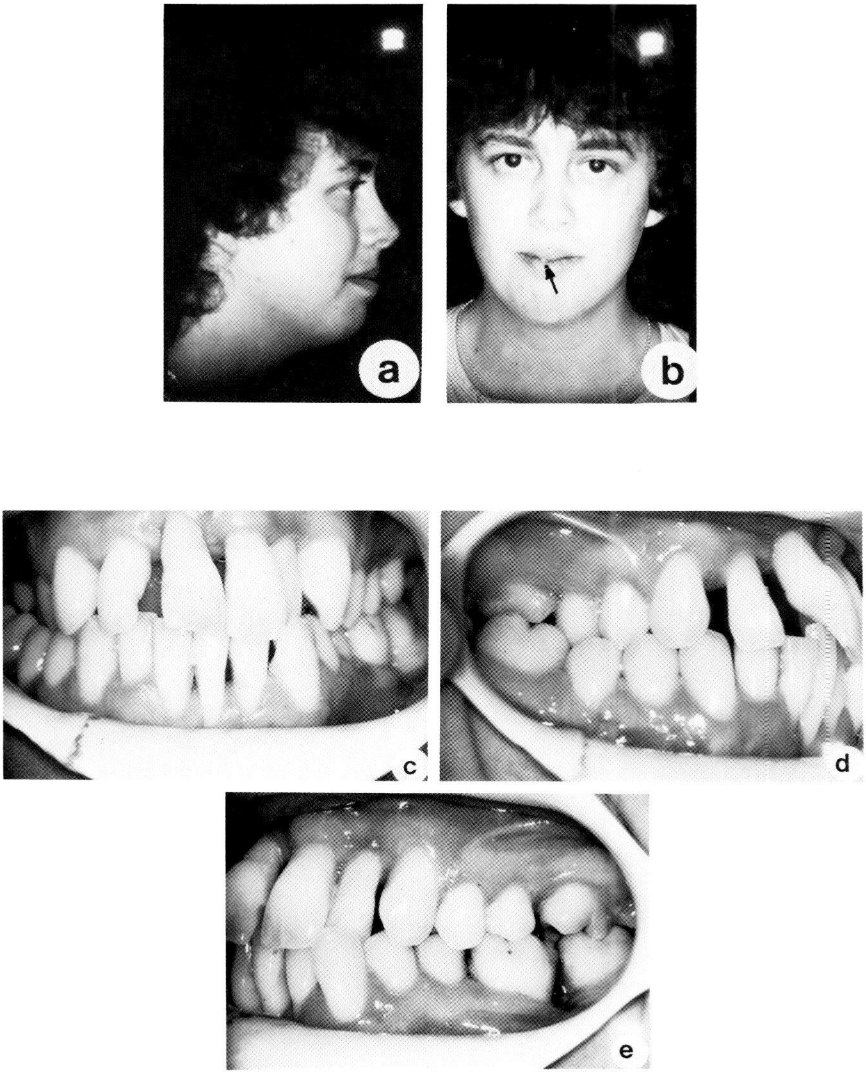

Figure 8. Case III. *A, B.* Extraoral view before treatment. The upper incisor is caught by the lower lip. *C-E.* Occlusal status before treatment. Pronounced irregularity is present.

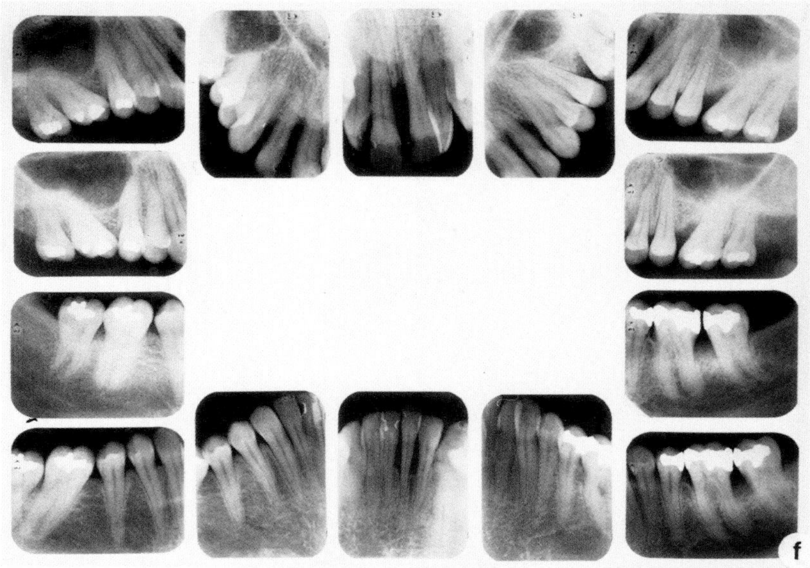

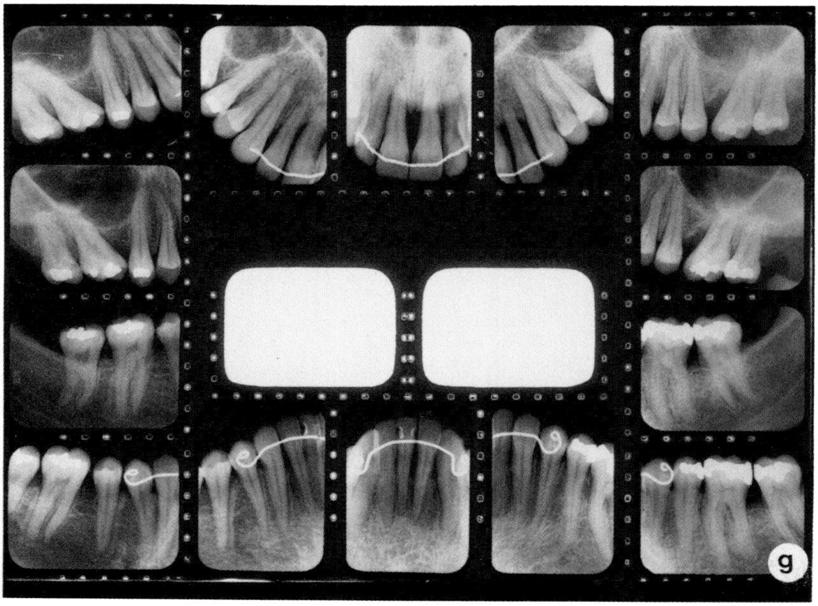

Figure 8, continued. *F.* Pretreatment periapical status. Note the marked original bone loss and the missing cortical bone bordering the alveolar process. *G.* Post-treatment status. An improved bone level in the incisor region is apparent. The bone density is generally improved as a result of improved chewing function.

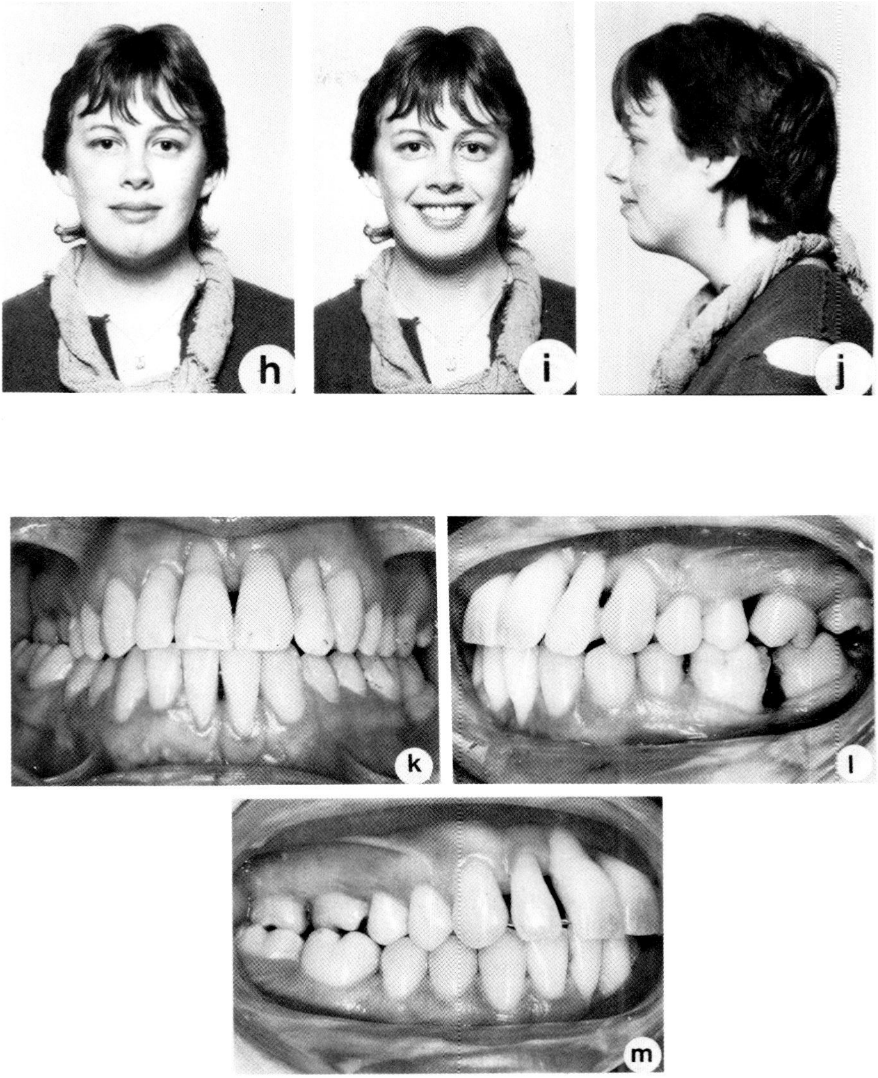

Figure 8, continued. *H-J.* Extraoral view post-treatment. The treatment result is stable and the bone density is further improved. *K-M.* Occlusal relationship post-treatment.

(2) extraction of all molars with subsequent resorption of the alveolar process, leaving a free-end saddle denture the only treatment possibility. With both of these problems, it is crucial that the tooth movement is carried out by bone modification and not through bone.

The re-establishment of a dental status in the posterior segments to allow the construction of fixed prosthetics is illustrated in the following two case presentations.

Selection of Biomechanics in Treating Tilted Second or Third Molars

Before any sort of appliance is applied to tilted molars, the appropriate force system should be determined. If a tooth is tilted into an extraction site, an uprighting and, often, mesial, movement is desirable, and vertical displacement is to be avoided. The optimal force in such a case would be equivalent to a mesially directed force applied apically to the center of resistance (CR), which in molars is localized slightly apically to the bifurcation (Burstone and Pryputniewicz, 1980). Since forces can only be applied to an attachment at the crown, a force system replacing a single force attaching apically to the CR is composed of a force and a moment.

The magnitude of the moment is calculated by multiplying the force by the perpendicular distance from the CR to the desired point of force application. If the moment is generated through a lever arm, the force system invariably produces extrusion of the molar, and in case of exaggerated forces, a vertical defect mesially, due to insufficient apposition at the marginal area where stretching of the periodontal fibers is most pronounced. An intrusion of the anchorage teeth can occur simultaneously, resulting in a deepening of the curve of Spee. The only way to avoid producing these vertical forces is to add an equivalent alpha moment to the anterior anchorage unit (Fig. 9). The alpha and beta moments would then neutralize the vertical forces corresponding to a geometry six defined in relation to the ideal arch (Burstone and Koenig, 1974). Since the moment on the anchorage teeth is undesirable, its effect should be minimized by joining as many teeth as possible in the anchorage group and by using the occlusal forces as a neutralizer.

If an uprighting moment and an active intrusion force of the molars are desired, the beta moment should be smaller than the alpha moment; the resulting extrusion force would then act in the anterior segment (Melsen et al., 1987*b*). The latter can, on the other hand, be prevented or minimized if spread over a large anchorage block, and thereby neutralized

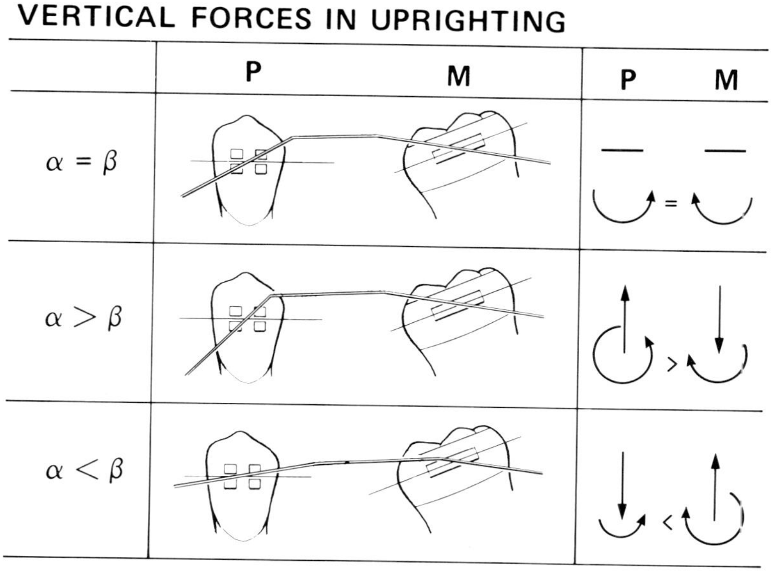

Figure 9. Molar-uprighting theory.

by occlusal forces. In order to distribute occlusal forces most equally and to let occlusion counteract the uprighting movement of the molars, an occlusal splint can be used on the part of the dental arch not involved in treatment, e.g., the anterior segment from the right to the left second premolar. This splint should be produced in an articulator, and have an occlusal profile giving the patient a sensation of a firm occlusion, and allow chewing with the splint in place. The splint may be removable, and if cemented must be very thin, adding to comfort without reducing the fracture risk. In patients where the occlusion is stable in the anterior segment, a splint may not be necessary, and the anchorage segment can be established as suggested by Roberts and colleagues (1982).

Case IV (Fig. 10)

A 36-year-old man, who had a very severe malocclusion with non-occlusion on the left side, experienced early extraction of both first and second permanent molars; the third molar was placed almost horizontally (Fig. 10*A*). The only chance of establishing a stable occlusion and eliminating the eventual need for a removable denture was to upright, intrude and move the third molar mesially.

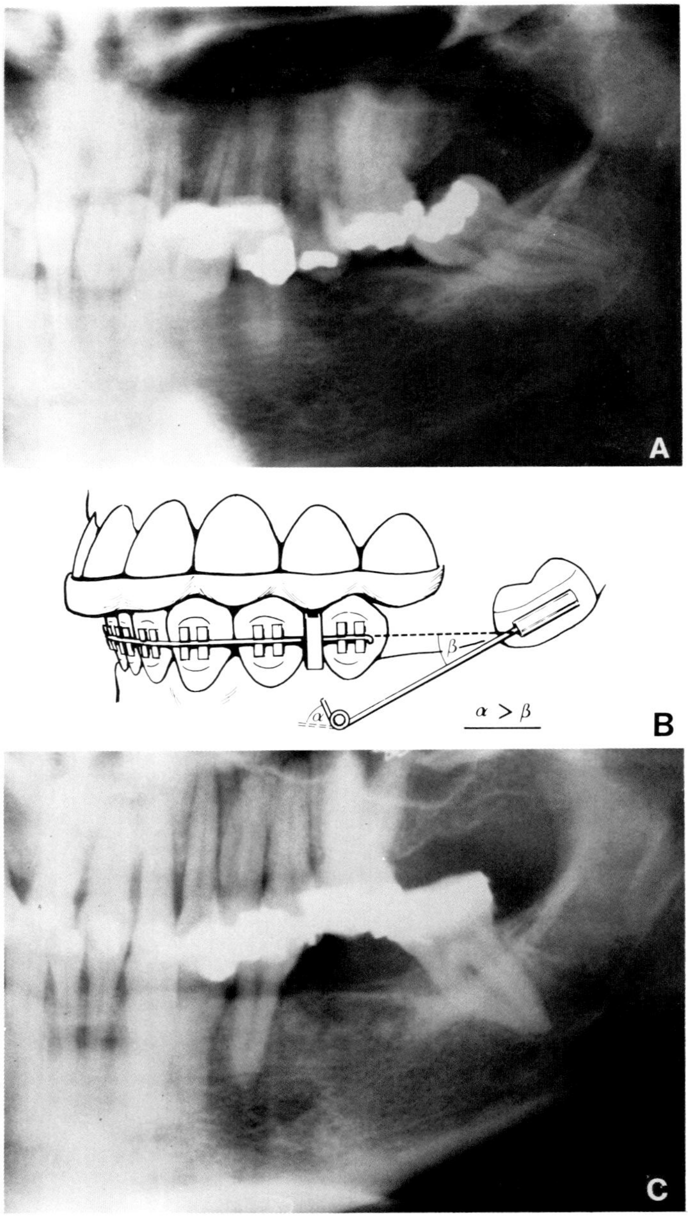

Figure 10. Case IV. *A*. Radiograph before treatment. *B*. Appliance design. *C*. Radiograph taken after treatment.

In this case the desirable force system was determined to be equivalent to one force applied apically to the center of resistance in a mesio-apical direction. The treatment was initiated during a period following a surgical maxillary impaction, when the patient was wearing a maxillary splint fixed by two infra-orbital wires. The uprighting spring was adjusted so that the alpha moment was 30% greater than the beta moment, producing approximately 20-30 g of intrusive force on the molars and a corresponding extrusive force on the premolars. Extrusion of the premolars was minimized through the above-mentioned splint (Fig. 10*B*). Following six weeks of maxillary fixation, the patient's splint was removed and was used as a removable retainer during the following 13 months of treatment. At this time the uprighting spring was again exchanged with a T-loop (Burstone, 1983), a protraction spring with a small beta and a bigger alpha moment. The situation at the end of treatment is shown in Fig. 10*C*.

Selection of Biomechanics in Cases of Extraction of All Molars: Case V (Fig. 11)

A 53-year-old woman was referred for orthodontic treatment by a dental school periodontal department. She had received comprehensive periodontal treatment, including a flap operation in the upper jaw. This was, however, not sufficient to obtain a satisfactory dentition and to stop the aggravation of her malocclusion. She reported that following extraction of the lower molars and insertion of a removable lower denture, the upper front teeth had started to drift forward and general diastemata had developed, along with a deep bite. The progressing atrophy of the alveolar processes had led to the necessity for underlining the denture a number of times, and she reported a feeling of fatigue in the temporofacial muscles. Her wish was to regain a stable occlusion and to eliminate anterior diastemata in the upper jaw.

Clinical Examination

Dental Status. In the upper jaw, both left first premolars had been extracted and replaced by a bridge. In the right side, the second premolar had been extracted and the space was nearly closed due to mesial rotation and migration of tooth number 16. In the lower jaw, only teeth 34 to 44 were present. The overjet was 13 mm, the overbite 8 mm.

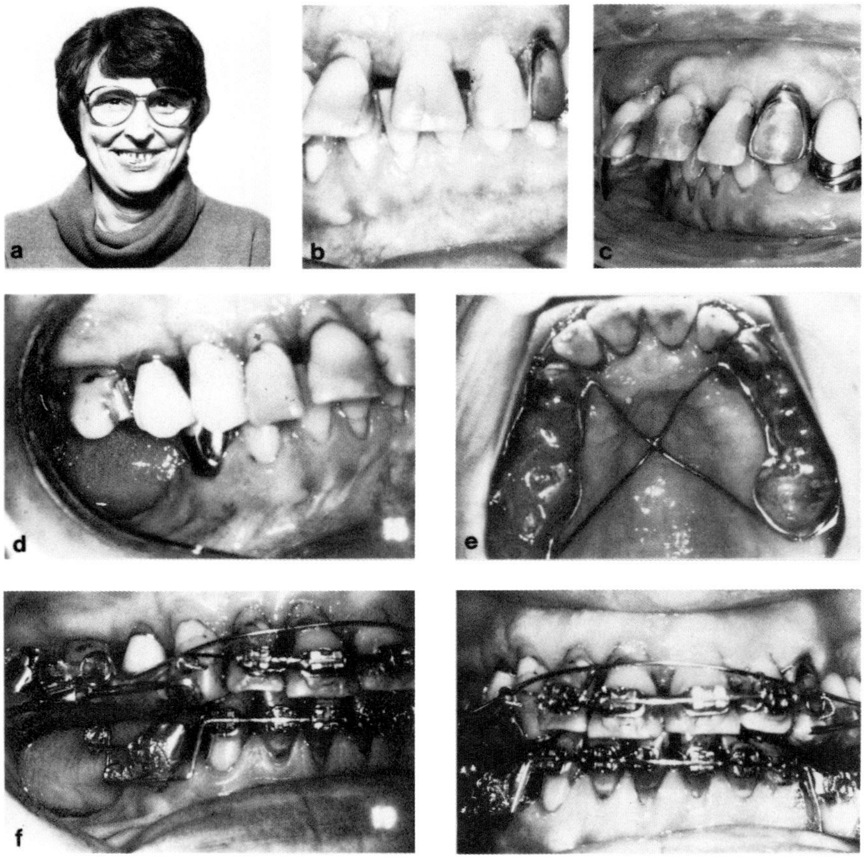

Figure 11. Case V. *A.* Extraoral photo taken prior to treatment. The upper incisors were caught by the lower lip during function. *B-D.* Intraoral status before treatment. There was pronounced spacing of the upper incisors, a deep overbite and an increased overjet. The lower second premolars and all molars were missing. The alveolar process was totally atrophic. *E.* The anchorage consisted of a splint into which the wires crossing the palate and serving as a base for the brackets were embedded. *F,G.* The appliance used for intrusion and retraction of incisors was a base arch with a point of force application distal to the laterals. During intrusion the stable segment connecting the incisors was bent in a curvature activation when forces from the base arch were applied to the extreme ends of the segment. Thereby a moment approximating the roots of the incisors was created. The crowns were simultaneously moved together by means of a power chain to the attachment. In the lower jaw, a loop was constructed delivering the moment to force ratio required for translation of the first premolars distally.

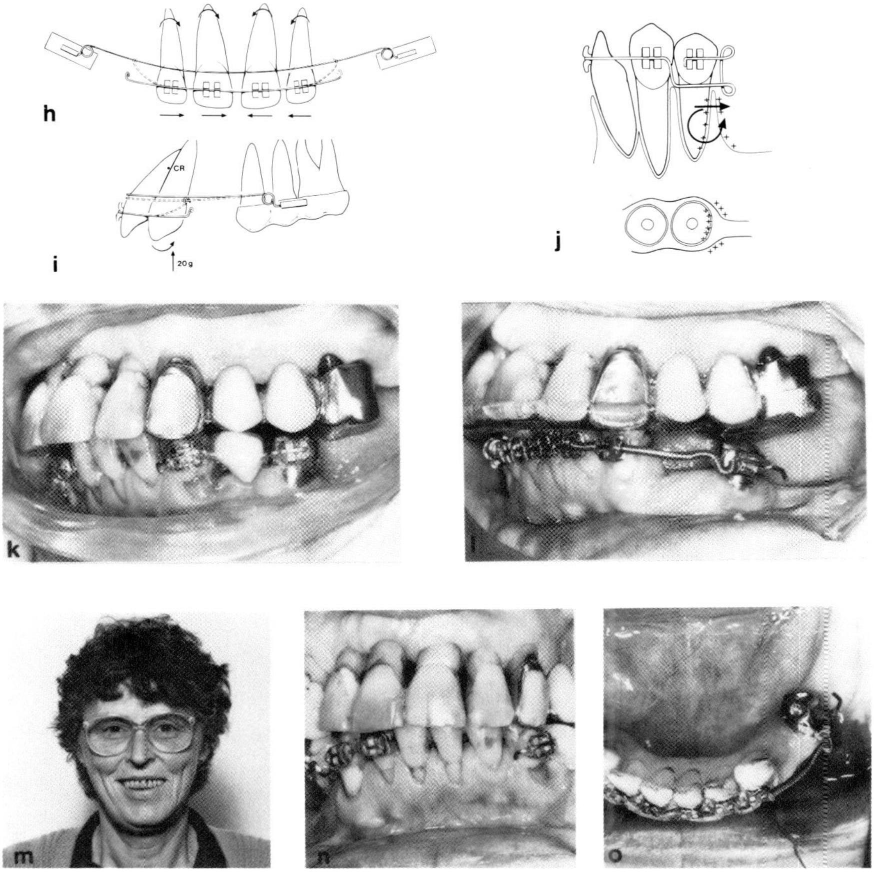

Figure 11, continued. *H, I.* Schematic drawing of the base arch in a frontal *(H)*, and a sagittal view *(I)*, showing how the moments bringing the incisor roots together were generated. *J.* Schematic drawing of the spring used for distal translation of the premolars using the anterior segment as anchorage. *K-O.* Post-treatment status. The overbite and overjet has been reduced through intrusion and retraction of upper incisor and proclination of the lower incisors. The right premolar has been translated distally to allow for fixed restoration. The left premolar exhibited a root fracture and was extruded in order to bring the fracture line above the gingival margin. This root will be moved distally following healing.

Periodontal Status. There was a general bone loss of 20 to 30%. The alveolar process was completely atrophic distal to the premolars.

Functional Status. The excessively spaced and elongated incisors were caught by the lower lip during swallowing and speech. The pterygoid and temporalis muscles were tender on palpation. The cephalometric analysis confirmed that the etiology of the deep bite was overeruption of the upper incisors due to lack of interincisal contact (and insufficient bone support).

Treatment Objective

To establish a mandibular position where the patient was free of muscular symptoms, the diastemata, the deep bite and the protruding spread incisors were to be treated by intrusion, retraction and retroclination of the upper incisors. The lower incisors should, in order to meet the requirements of a stable incisal relationship, be proclined slightly. Stabilization of the occlusion was to be attempted by extension of the periodontally supported part of the occlusion through distal translation of the first lower bicuspids. The mucosa-supported removable lower denture could thereby be replaced by bridges.

Appliances

Two splint segments were fitted in the maxillary side segments and joined by a cross across the palate. The cemented splint was equilibrated and used to determine the optimal mandibular position. In the upper jaw, the anterior teeth were joined with 0.017 x 0.025 inch stainless steel wire extending laterally to the canine region, ending in a small helix which was localized distal to the center of resistance of the total anterior block of teeth. The intrusive forces were produced by means of a base arch *ad modum* Burstone (1977). The point of force application was the helix of the anterior segment, and the force level was 10-15 g per tooth.

The tooth movement obtained was a combination of an intrusion and distal tipping. Since the wire of the anterior segment was long and the point of force application at the extreme end, the anterior arch section bent into a curvature which produced a bending moment bringing the roots together (Fig. 11). A power chain added a horizontal force at the level of the brackets, thus resulting in a translation of the incisors towards the midline.

In the lower jaw, a modified rectangular loop was used for bodily movement of the premolars distally. The necessary moment was equilibrated in the anchorage group with buccal root torque of the lower incisors (Fig. 11*J*).

Result

The elongated and spaced incisors had been intruded and retruded. Increased pocket depth developed during treatment, probably as a result of the accumulation of mucosa on the lingual side of the incisors. A second periodontal surgery was therefore necessary. Interincisal contact was established, and in the lower jaw the alveolar process was rebuilt and distal movement of the premolars was produced. Following treatment, the patient was referred back to the dentist for further reconstruction. (Fig. 11*K-O*).

In relation to the second category of problem involved in this case, i.e., distal displacement of premolar into an edentulous area and atrophia of the alveolar process, it is essential that the stress distribution is totally under control. It is desirable to displace the premolars distally, making it possible to prepare for a bridge in the side segment to provide the upper teeth with the necessary occlusal contacts. If the premolars are just tipped distally, the greatest force will develop marginally and the marginal bone will gradually disappear through a resorption, leading to apical displacement of the marginal bone level. If, on the other hand, a spring is used to deliver a moment to force ratio that will displace the root in front of the crown, a gradual reconstruction of the alveolar process will be produced.

CONCLUSION

1. Treatment of a degenerating dentition means much more to the patient than just re-establishment of the chewing apparatus. Treatment of the degenerating dentition must be handled through an interdisciplinary approach.
2. Patients' treatment expectations should be in agreement with reality.
3. The orthodontic treatment must be planned with special regard to anchorage and vertical control.
4. The force systems should be adapted to the bone density and the marginal bone level.

5. Only the segmented arch offers these necessary options. Maintenance of the post-treatment result must be understood and accepted by the patient.

REFERENCES

Briedenhann, S.J. and J.F. van Reenen. Tooth extraction and tooth mutilating practices amongst the Herero-speaking peoples of South West Africa (Namibia). J. Dent. Assoc. S. Africa *40:*531-536, 1985.

Burstone, C.J. The rationale of the segmented arch. Am. J. Orthod. *48:*805-822, 1962.

Burstone, C.J. Deep overbite correction by intrusion. Am. J. Orthod. *72:*1-22, 1977.

Burstone, C.J. The segmented approach to space closure. Am. J. Orthod. *82:*361-377, 1982.

Burstone, C.J. Application of bioengineering to clinical orthodontics. In: *Orthodontics: Current Principles and Techniques.* T.M. Graber and B.F. Swann (Eds.), C.V. Mosby Co., St. Louis, 1985.

Burstone, C.J. and H.A. Koenig. Force systems from an ideal arch. Am. J. Orthod. *65:*270-289, 1974.

Burstone, C.J. and H.A. Koenig. Creative wire bending. The force system from step and "V" bends. Am. J. Orthod. *93:*59-63, 1988.

Burstone, C.J. and R.J. Pryputniewicz. Holographic determination of centers of rotation produced by orthodontic forces. Am. J. Orthod. *77:*396-409, 1980.

Fontenelle, A. Orthodontie à linguales: Une autre approche. Orthod. Fr. *57:*541-557, 1986.

Freud, S. *Interpretation of Dreams.* New York, Buccaneer Books, 1983.

Goldstein, R. Orthodontics and full mouth reconstruction. Paper read before the Greater N.Y. Academy of Prosthodontics, 1968.

Jung, C.G. *Dream Analysis: Notes of the Seminar Given in 1928-30.* Routledge & Kegan Paul, London, 1984.

Jung, C.G. *Dreams.* Routledge & Kegan Paul, London, 1982.

Lindhe, J. *Textbook of Clinical Periodontology.* Munksgaard, Copenhagen, 1983.

Marcotte, M.R. The use of the occlusogram in planning orthodontic treatment. Am. J. Orthod. *69:*655-677, 1976.

Melsen, B. *Treatment Problems in Adult Patients.* Nederlandse Vereniging voor Orthodontische Studie, Noordwijkerhout, 1980.

Melsen, B. Mise au point sur l'orthodontie de l'adulte. Quelles en sont les limites? Rev. Orthop. Dentofac. *20:*537-66, 1986.

Melsen, B. Adult orthodontics factors differentiating the selection of biomechanics in growing and adult individuals. Int. J. Adult Orthod. Orthognath. Surg., 1988, in press.

Melsen, B., N. Hørup and S. Terp. Factors of importance for maintenance of teeth. Comm. Dent. Health *4:*11-25, 1987*a*.

Melsen, B., S. Williams and F. Ronay. Differenzierte Kraftsysteme zur Aufrichtung von Molaren. Z. Stomatol. *84:*185-193, 1987*b*.

Melsen, B., N. Agerbæk and G. Markenstam. Intrusion of incisors in adult patients with marginal bone loss. Am. J. Orthod., 1988*a*, in press.

Melsen, B., N. Agerbæk, J. Eriksen and S. Terp. New attachment through periodontal treatment and orthodontic intrusion. Am. J. Orthod., 1988*b*, in press.

Melsen, F. Histomorphometric analyses of iliac bone in normal and pathological condition. Master's thesis, Aarhus University, 1978.

Musich, D. Assessment and description of the treatment needs of adult patients evaluated for orthodontic therapy II characteristics of the dual provider group. Int. J. Adult Orthod. Orthognath. Surg. *1:*101-117, 1986*a.*

Musich, D. Assessment and description of the treatment needs of adult patients for orthodontic therapy. III. Characteristic of the multiple provider group. Int. J. Adult Orthod. Orthognath. Surg. *4:*251-274, 1986*b.*

Møller, E. The myogenic factor in headache and facial pain. In: *Oral-Facial Sensory and Motor Functions.* Y. Kawamura and R. Dubner (Eds.), Quintessence, Tokyo, 1981.

Møller, E. and M. Bakke. Malocclusion morphologique et fonctionelle. Orthod. Fr. *57:*477-560, 1986.

Picton, D.C.A. The effect of external forces on the periodontium. In: *Biology of the Periodontium.* A.H. Melchior and W.H. Boween (Eds.), Academic Press, London, 1969.

Ramfjörd, S.P. and M.M. Ash. *Periodontology and Periodontics.* W.B. Saunders Co., Philadelphia, 1979.

Roberts, W., F. Chacker and C.J. Burstone. A segmented approach to mandibular molar uprighting. Am. J. Orthod. *81:*177-184, 1982.

Ronay, F., B. Melsen, W. Kleinert and C.J. Burstone *et al.* Force system developed by "V"-bends in an elastic orthodontic wire. Am. J. Orthod., 1988, in press.

Schei, O., J. Waerhaug, A. Lovdal and A. Arnulf. Alveolar bone loss as related to oral hygiene and age. J. Periodont. *26:*7-16, 1959.

Seide, L.J. Adult orthodontics. J. Prosthet. Dent. *24:*83-93, 1976.

Thurow, R.C. Cranio-maxillary orthopedic correction with en masse dental control. Am. J. Orthod. *68:*601-624, 1975.

Vanarsdall, R.L. and D.R. Musich. Adult orthodontics: Diagnosis and treatment. In: *Orthodontics: Current Principles and Techniques.* T.M. Graber and B.F. Swann (Eds.), The C.V. Mosby Company, St. Louis, 1985.

van Reenen, J.F. Tooth mutilation amongst the peoples of Kavango and Bushmanland, South West Africa (Namibia). J. Dent. Assoc. S. Afr. *33(4):*205-218, 1978.

van Reenen, J.F. and S.J. Briedenhann. Further observations on the tooth mutilating practices of Vassekela and Kung Bushmen. J. Dent. Assoc. S. Afr. *41:*557-562, 1986.

TEMPOROMANDIBULAR DISORDERS IN THE AGED

Christian S. Stohler

INTRODUCTION

There are a number of facial pain conditions that demonstrate an increased incidence with increasing age. For example, the onset of tic douloureux (idiopathic trigeminal neuralgia) occurs most often between 40 and 70 years of age (Heyck, 1981). Sphenopalatine and glossopharyngeal neuralgia, carotidynia, and Eagle's syndrome (stylohyoid syndrome) are known as diseases of the middle age population; postherpetic neuralgia and glossodynia are found primarily in the middle age group and the elderly (Eversole, 1978). In addition, the skeleton undergoes alterations with age which may be regarded either as inevitable consequences of use, as pathologic, or as a combination thereof. Such skeletal changes, particularly of the cervical spine, may also give rise to facial pain and headache.

However, other facial pain and headache such as the classic and common migraine show a distinct drop in incidence after the age of 30. In fact, the occurrence of first migraines after the age of 50 is mostly associated with some vascular or other organic disease. Cluster headaches first occur at any age between 10 and 60 (Heyck, 1981); only about 10% occur for the first time above age 50 (Kudrow, 1980). A first appearance of tension headache in elderly persons was found in only 3% of 466 patients given that diagnosis (Lance *et al.,* 1965). Pain associated with acute infection of the paranasal sinuses is also rare in the aged (Agate, 1986).

The number of publications in the field of aging, gerontology and geriatrics has grown enormously over the past decade. However, the subject of temporomandibular disorders in the elderly has not received great attention. The skeletal and dental changes associated with aging, for example, neglected dentitions and ill-fitting dentures that often replace the lost dentition, lead one to expect an increasing incidence of temporomandibular (TM) disorders with increasing age. The present paper reviews the literature with respect to the aging of the masticatory apparatus and its relationship to etiological and epidemiological aspects of TM disorders.

DEFINITIONS

The question arises as to when a subject may be designated "aged" or "elderly." It has been suggested that the term "the aging" is to be used for subjects between 68 and 75 years of age. Similarly, the term "the elderly" is applied to those between 76 and 85 years of age (Watkin, 1982). However, in the context of this paper, these terms are used in the conventional generic sense without reference to specific age groups.

Observable phenomena are referred to as "age-associated" or "age-correlated" in so far as they occur more frequently in subjects above a certain age, but they themselves cannot be regarded as "age-related" or "age-induced" (Hall, 1984), as the latter imply primary causal effects.

THE AGING MASTICATORY APPARATUS

The limited research attention paid in the dental field to issues related to aging of the masticatory apparatus has most recently (1987) been addressed by the National Institute of Dental Research and the Veterans Administration, which called for proposals for geriatric centers. Much of the available material on the subject is based on observations made in body systems other than the masticatory apparatus. With respect to TM disorders, the masticatory system is capable of generating only a very limited number of signs and symptoms. Symptoms include pain, stiffness, and complaints of impaired function or of a systemic nature; signs are tenderness, limited range of motion and joint sounds. The question is whether or not aging increases the likelihood that these disease descriptors will occur. Later in this paper, age-associated and age-induced changes in sensory and motor function, including aging of mandibular and condylar cartilage, will be discussed in as far as they relate to temporomandibular disorders.

Pain in the Aging

Excellent reviews of the neurophysiological (Storey, 1983; Sessle, 1987*a,b*) and psychological aspects of pain in general (Rugh, 1987) have recently been published. Data on pain specifically in the aging are less clear. It is generally accepted that the elderly are reticent about reporting pain. In addition, pains "here and there" are often ignored by older people because of other, more demanding health problems. Notable in this context is the fact of a reduced pain tolerance in patients with TM disorders (Molin *et al.*, 1973). There is evidence that the pain threshold changes as individuals age. In fact, the threshold for cutaneous pricking pain, tested by means of a thermal algometer, increases progressively with increasing age as established on representative samples of 18 to 28-year-old (N=258) and 50 to 90-year-old subjects (N=267) (Procacci *et al.*, 1985). The cutaneous heat threshold decreases approximately 10 to 20% with age (Chapman and Jones, 1944; Schluderman and Zubeck, 1952; Sherman and Robillard, 1964; Mumford, 1968; Harkins and Warner, 1980), which strongly suggests reduced pain sensitivity in the elderly. However, this finding is limited to acute pain and may not be true for chronic pain. Rather than a sharp, localized pain, TM disorders are most frequently associated with dull, diffuse aching (Bell, 1985). However, little information is available with regard to the deep somatic pain threshold and its relationship to age. A decreased achilles tendon pain tolerance with age (Woodrow *et al.,* 1972) suggests increased deep somatic pain sensitivity in the elderly. Since the perception of the deep somatic pain is modulated by endogenous pain suppressive mechanisms, any age-related deficiency of serotonin and enkephalin could explain this finding.

A recent thesis has drawn renewed attention to the association of headaches and TM disorders (Forssell, 1985). Evidence of such an association has been noted in a number of epidemiological studies (Agerberg and Carlsson, 1973, 1975; Helkimo, 1974*c*; Hansson and Nilner, 1975; Molin *et al.,* 1976; Heloe and Heloe, 1979; Solberg *et al.,* 1979; Ingervall *et al.,* 1980). Changes in headache and mandibular dysfunction after occlusal treatment have been documented longitudinally over a time span of 2.5 years (Magnusson and Carlsson, 1983). Alleviation of headache symptoms has been reported in association with successful treatment of TM disorders (Agerberg and Carlsson, 1974). Magnusson (1981) suggested that headaches should be regarded as a symptom of TM disorders. As far as the aged are concerned, headaches generally decrease in frequency with increasing age (Waters, 1974; Newland *et al.,* 1978). Only the headaches attributable to cerebrovascular disease, cervical osteoarthritis and giant cell arteritis are clearly more frequent with age (Hammerstad, 1985).

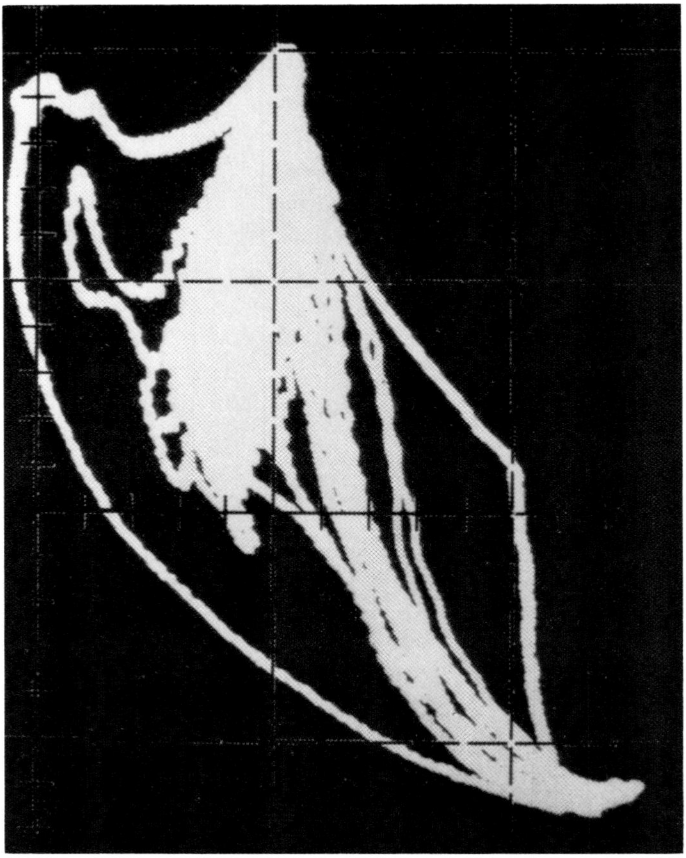

Figure 1. Envelope of mandibular motion as projected in the sagittal plane. Within the boundaries of the envelope, maximum open-close and chewing movements are displayed. Note that the chewing movements are well within the envelope of motion.

The Aging Motor System

There is a significant reduction in muscle strength directly related to age (Aniansson *et al.,* 1978; Larsson *et al.,* 1978; Aniansson, 1980; Aniansson *et al.,* 1981; Clarkson *et al.,* 1981). The question of whether these effects are truly age-related or are influenced by other factors, such as motivation, remains to be answered. Isometric and isotonic quadriceps strength increases between 10 to 14 years of age and 20 to 29 years of age, remains unchanged until 40 to 49 years of age, and then gradually declines (Larsson, 1978). However, this can only be explained in part by age-related effects in the skeletal musculature, which decreases relative to total body weight with increasing age (MacLennan *et al.,* 1980). The cause of muscle weakness is probably multifactorial (Cheshire and Cumming, 1985). Denervation in the quadriceps of healthy 78 to 81-year-old subjects has been reported (Grimby *et al.,* 1982). The specific age-related changes in the muscle tissue, as documented in the rat, include (1) a decrease in the number of type IIa muscle fibers, and (2) a decrease in the diameter of type IIb muscle fibers (McCarter, 1978). Both types are regarded as fast twitch fibers and are primarily recruited in phasic activity. Type IIa is considered to be resistant to fatigue, and type IIb as rapidly fatiguing (Burke *et al.,* 1973). Approximately 50 to 60% of the human masseter muscle is of the fast, fatigable fiber type (Ringqvist, 1971, 1973). However, a more detailed analysis in rhesus monkeys revealed marked differences in fiber composition between different parts of the masseter and also with respect to sex (Maxwell *et al.,* 1979).

Age-related effects in the central nervous system include a decrease in the number of motor fibers of about 5% per decade (Gutmann, 1977), and a 20% decrease in nerve impulse conduction velocity between the ages of 35 and 85 years (Strehler, 1976).

As a sign of decline in motor function in the masticatory system in particular, the Baltimore Longitudinal Study of Aging reported a higher incidence of labial drool of saliva or reduced tongue stability in old age (Baum, 1979). In view of the decreased tissue mobility associated with the well-documented age-related changes in extracellular polymers, the correlation between maximum mouth opening and age, however, is relatively weak (Behjou and Stohler, 1988). Reports of the average maximum mouth opening range from 43-59 mm, with values for females in general being slightly smaller (Posselt, 1952; Travell, 1960; Nevakari, 1960; Agerberg, 1974*b*; Bosman, 1974; Solberg *et al.,* 1979; Ogura *et al.,* 1985). Due to the fact that the range of mandibular movement needed for chewing constitutes only about 50% or less of the total mandibular mobility range, age-related stiffness or rigidity is not of importance to the chewing function in old age (Fig. 1). Similarly, in the absence of masticatory dysfunction, the maximum available bite force exceeds that needed for chewing (Bates *et al.,* 1975), so that the age-related deficit usually does not become apparent. However, of particular importance in the elderly are drug-induced neuromuscular effects. Mandibular tremor and rigidity can be associated with high doses of phenothiazine (Kline, 1968). Drug-induced myopathy, particularly inflammatory myopathy, muscle cramps, fasciculations, muscle aches, or stiffness, are observed with medications widely used in the aged, such as penicillamine, lithium, procainamide, hydralazine and others (Argov and Mastaglia, 1979; Hudgson, 1982). It should be emphasized, however, that what has been documented for the limb musculature does not necessarily apply for the masticatory system as well (Vanderspek *et al.,* 1988).

Age-Related Functional Deficit

Aging is apparent throughout life, but is more noticeable in the post-reproductive period (Hall, 1984). Age-related changes of performance were recently reviewed by Welford (1985). In general, the aged organism shows a decrease in physiologic function with increasing age. The increased prevalence of labial drool of saliva and reduced tongue stability in old age are examples of this decrease in function (Baum, 1979). The frequency of swallowing dysfunctions is greater in middle-aged and older subjects than in younger ones. This is of particular importance in light of laryngeal food spills and their potentially disastrous consequences (Bosma, 1976; Baum, 1979). It is not understood if these age-related findings reflect changes in the sensory system, the motor system, or both. In individuals for whom normal functional demands can be met, the age-related deficit is brought out only when the system is stressed. For example, the normal walking pace changes little with age; on the other hand, the maximum walking pace declines appreciably (Cunningham *et al.,* 1982). However, if the functional demands can no longer be met, coping efforts and compensatory strategies will be put into effect. For example, difficulty in chewing may be minimized by cutting foods into smaller pieces, avoiding certain foods, exercising a strong masticatory lateral preference, careful bolus placement, frequent bolus reshaping and, occasionally, conscious control over the otherwise involuntary act of chewing. Any discomfort from dentures or difficulty keeping them in place when eating or speaking is likely to disrupt the smooth programming of the actions involved and, on occasion, will capture conscious attention (Welford, 1979). Denture wearers with impaired retention and stability of the lower prostheses show an increased use of the lower lip and mentalis muscle (Tallgren, 1963), which is considered a coping strategy to deal with the ill-fitting denture. Notable in this context is also the significantly reduced production of parotid saliva in the elderly (Franks and Hedegard, 1973).

The Aging Mandible and Condylar Cartilage

Since many joint diseases are chronic, there is a steady cumulative effect on their prevalence with age. In fact, 80% of the population experiences some type of rheumatological disorder by the time of retirement (Kolodny and Klipper, 1976). This means that the frequency of this type of condition is age-associated because the likelihood of the disease to manifest itself is greater if more time is available. As documented in a study using 100 subjects between 18 and 67 years of age, normal remodeling of the temporal and mandibular components of the TMJ occurs predominantly between 18 and 25 years of age, after which its influence appears to be less prominent (Mongini, 1972).

Insofar as the articular surfaces are concerned, the collagen matrix responsible for the resiliency of the articular tissues is of particular importance. The relative stability, with increasing age, of the amount and proportion of glycosaminoglycans (the proteoglycan component associated with the retention of extracellular fluid) in the joints implies that mechanical loading, rather than age, is the principal variable (Mohl, 1988). The changes of collagen associated with aging in the mandible, and in aging articular cartilage in general, have recently been reviewed in great detail (Gardner and O'Connor, 1985; Shikata *et al.,* 1987).

RISK FACTORS FOR TM DISORDERS DURING AGING

There is little agreement as to what causes TM disorders (Zarb and Mohl, 1988). Most authors support a multifactorial model, however, with varying emphasis on the role of occlusal, psychophysiological, biomechanical, muscular and neuromuscular factors. In this section, risk factors are reviewed for possible differences in the aged.

The Aging Occlusion

A neglected dentition, particularly loss of teeth, is associated with the aged. Zarb and Thompson (1975) claimed that a neglected dentition with lack of, or incorrect, prosthodontic rehabilitation can bring about temporomandibular joint dysfunction. Inappropriate use of the masticatory apparatus, such as with incorrect or deficient prosthodontic treatment, has been suggested to predispose to degenerative joint disease at any age; however, this is more likely in the aged. In fact, the incidence of osteoarthrosis is influenced by many factors other than age, including heredity, previous joint disease and trauma, metabolic factors, and diet (Grahame, 1985). A weak correlation between tooth loss and TMJ arthrosis has been found (Oberg *et al.,* 1971). Comparing dental status in terms of tooth loss between symptomatic and asymptomatic subjects, Franks (1968) and Helkimo (1974*b*) reported less favorable conditions in symptomatic subjects. However, Agerberg and Carlsson (1975) as well as Molin and colleagues (1976) did not observe a difference between groups as far as tooth loss is concerned. Thomson (1971) could not find any significant difference in posterior support between 100 patients with TM disorders and a similar number of control subjects.

With respect to the future, there will always be a certain percentage of edentulous subjects in any population; however, the elderly will, in general, retain most of a functional natural dentition. The question of whether this will affect the future prevalence and incidence of TM disorders in the aged remains speculative at this time. Notable in this context is the fact that maximum bite force in dentate subjects is about five to six times greater than in denture wearers (Haraldsson *et al.,* 1979).

In addition to the factor of tooth loss, particular occlusal factors may be of importance in the development of TM disorders. A number of morphologically-defined occlusal configurations were studied in order to investigate whether their frequency was particularly high in symptomatic subjects. However, only weak correlations between certain of these occlusal conditions and signs and symptoms of TM disorders have been found in epidemiological investigations (Molin *et al.,* 1976; Solberg *et al.,* 1979; Ingervall *et al.,* 1980; Egermark-Eriksson, 1982; Egermark-Eriksson *et al.,* 1983) and studies in clinical material (Geering, 1974; Maruyama *et al.,* 1982; DeBoever and Adriaens, 1983). Such weak correlations do not support the existence of a causal effect for occlusal factors in TM disorders. Nevertheless, it is often assumed by clinicians that such cause-effect relationships clearly exist. The individual occlusion should be characterized by its influence on the oral motor behavior, rather than by morphologic description of occlusal interferences. Due to the fact that the available data are far from being conclusive in the general population, it is inappropriate to discuss possible age-specific effects of occlusal interferences.

Psychophysiological Factors in the Aged

Two recent, excellent reviews (Hodgson and Jolley, 1985; Post, 1985) give a comprehensive view of the emotional state of the elderly. Insofar as emotional factors are concerned, stress is considered a prime factor in the etiology of TM disorders. The question arises whether the elderly, as a group, are particularly stressed or adapt to stress differently than younger subjects. Empirical studies suggest that differences exist, e.g., the loss of a spouse later as opposed to earlier in life is somewhat different because of anticipatory socialization (Tobin, 1985). However, the available information is too limited to warrant a meaningful discussion of this etiological factor in the development of TM disorders in the aged.

Many older individuals undergo a period characterized by depressive complaints (Stenback *et al.,* 1979; Gurland *et al.,* 1980; Blazer and Williams, 1980) or depressive preoccupations. This coincides with a transitional phase in life during which satisfactory adjustments to the status of the elderly are made (Gianturco and Busse, 1978). However, the prevalence of major depressions in the elderly is actually lower than at any other stage of adult life (Weissman and Myers, 1981). Since depressive states are believed to influence sensitivity to pain and willingness to tolerate pain (Rugh, 1987), this condition may occasionally be of importance as a possible factor in TM disorders.

Parafunction in the Aging

Parafunctional oral habits such as teeth grinding or clenching are very common. On occasion adverse effects such as excessive tooth wear and muscle hypertrophy are associated with these habits. There is evidence to support the notion that masticatory muscle pain and headaches can result from such activities.

The subject of nocturnal bruxism has most recently been reviewed by Rugh and Harlan (1988). Prevalence data are either based upon questionnaire information or clinical examinations. The existing epidemiological information has recently been summarized by Seligman and colleagues (1988). Data relative to parafunctional oral motor behavior in denture wearers, however, are scarce (Zarb, 1979). Nocturnal bruxism is clearly more frequent in children with brain defects (Lindqvist and Heijbel, 1974), subjects with emotional disturbances (Lindqvist, 1972), the mentally retarded (Richmond *et al.,* 1981), adults with tardive dyskinesia (a complication of long-term neuroleptic therapy characterized

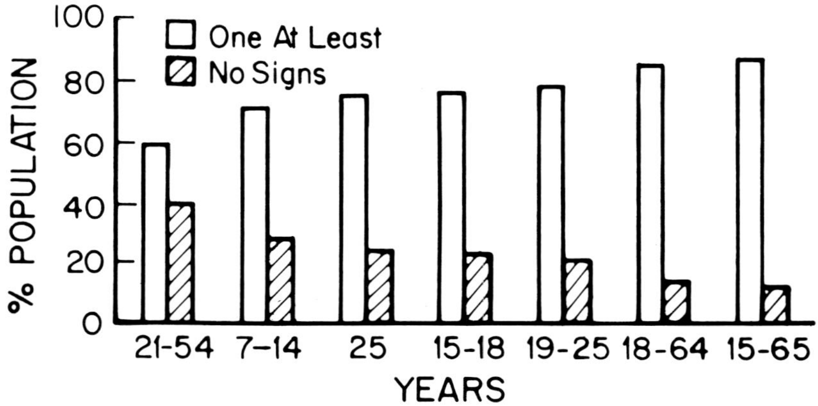

Figure 2. Prevalence of at least one or no sign of the classic triad in populations of specified age ranges. Results shown for each age range are from the following studies: Molin *et al.,* 1976 (21-54 yrs.); Nilner and Lassing, 1981 (7-14 yrs.); Heloe and Heloe, 1979 (25 yrs.); Nilner, 1981 (15-18 yrs.); Solberg *et al.,* 1979 (19-25 yrs.); Swanljung and Rantanen, 1979 (18-64 yrs.); Helkimo, 1974 (15-65 yrs.).

by involuntary movements of tongue, lips and facial musculature; Kamen, 1975), and alcoholics (Hartmann, 1979); it is found about equally in children and adults (Glaros, 1981). The reported prevalence of bruxism in adults ranges from 5.1 to 22.2% (Reding *et al.,* 1966; Meklas, 1971; Thompson *et al.,* 1972; Wigdorowicz-Makowerowa *et al.,* 1979; Rieder, 1977; Glaros, 1981) and from 11.6 to 15.1% in children (Reding *et al.,* 1966; Lindqvist, 1971). The prevalence of clenching has been reported in as many as 40% of the population studied (Ingervall *et al.,* 1980). Dental attrition is not associated with the presence or absence of TMJ clicking and masticatory muscle or joint tenderness (Seligman *et al.,* 1988). Attrition scores do not differ significantly between age groups, indicating that notable attrition, when present, often occurs early (Seligman *et al.,* 1988). Tardive dyskinesia, however, is particularly frequent between 50 and 70 years of age (Kamen, 1975). With increasing attention paid in dentistry to conditions found in older individuals, the extent of this problem in institutionalized patients, or, more generally, in older subjects without obvious neurologic deficiency, will become better defined.

Diurnal parafunctional oral habits can be found in every age group. These habits, however, are more commonly associated with younger children and include, e.g., thumb-sucking. No epidemiological studies of the incidence of diurnal parafunction in the aged have been conducted.

SYMPTOMATIC SUBJECTS AMONG THE ELDERLY

Epidemiology has contributed greatly to the discovery of possible causal relationships, particularly in infectious or vascular diseases. However, in the field of TM disorders, epidemiological research has raised many unanswered questions.

An excellent review of the literature critically examined the existing epidemiological data for TM disorders (Solberg, 1983). All of the available information is based on the cross-sectional assessment of the age effect with respect to signs and symptoms. Changes with age have traditionally been inferred from either the average differences observed between measurements made on groups of subjects of different ages, or from the regression on age of observations made on subjects distributed over the total age span who were measured at the same time (Shock, 1985). In the elderly, subjects with either (1) impaired range of mobility, (2) pain and tenderness of the temporomandibular joints or masticatory muscles, (3) temporomandibular joint sounds, or (4) combinations thereof are reported with similar frequency (Heloe, 1972; Heloe and Heloe, 1979; Swanljung and Rantanen, 1979), or slightly higher frequency than among the general population (Helkimo, 1974*a*; Lysell, 1977; Makila, 1979; Osterberg and Carlsson, 1979). About 20% of young adults are reported as asymptomatic (Solberg *et al.,* 1979), compared to 15% of the elderly (Osterberg and Carlsson, 1979).

The available data should be accepted with reservations with respect to the effect of age (Fig. 2). Epidemiological investigations up to this point have examined a group of subjects at one point in time, rather than following a cohort for a number of years. Validation of possible age-related effects has to be provided by longitudinal observation. The range within which epidemiological studies reported the prevalence of each element of the classic triad is given in Figure 3. However, whether or not these frequent signs or symptoms should be considered expression of normality, preclinical features, or manifestations of disease is not an-

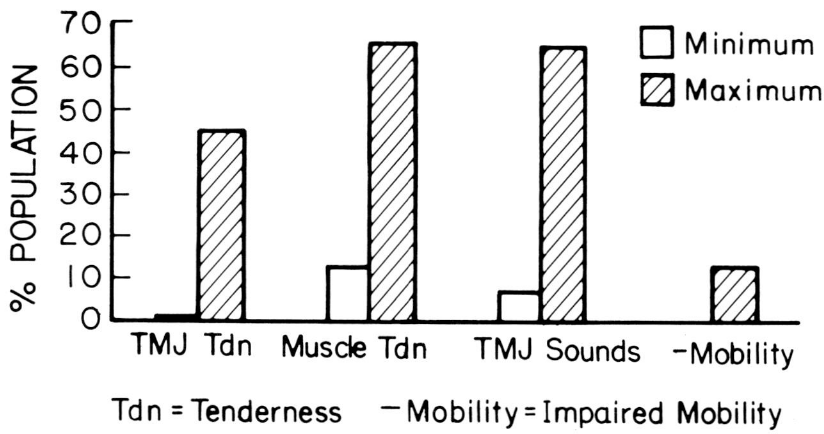

Figure 3. Range (min-max) within which epidemiological studies reported the prevalence of each of the elements of the classic triad.

swered by these investigations. The mere existence of loose disease descriptors with as yet unvalidated relationships to disease should not be confused with disease or treatment need.

TEMPOROMANDIBULAR DISORDERS IN THE AGED

The use of the all-inclusive term "TM disorders" is regarded as very limiting and the need to distinguish clinically identifiable subgroups has been recognized (Bell, 1983). The relationship of signs and symptoms as they relate to subgroups of TM disorders has not been the focus of epidemiological research up to this point. For example, crepitus, not muscle tenderness, nor impaired mandibular mobility, is the most reliable clinical sign of osteoarthrosis (Hansson and Nilner, 1975). However, myogenous pain and muscle tenderness are the primary characteristics of the acute masticatory muscle disorders (Bell, 1983). The fact that epidemiological studies report a high prevalence of signs and symptoms of TM disorders in general should not suggest that such disorders are a quasi-universal disease (Zarb and Mohl, 1988). Although signs and symptoms such as impaired range of mandibular mobility, tenderness of jaw musculature and joints, and joint sounds are widely accepted indicators of TM disorders, the significance of epidemiological findings in terms of the true pathology are far from clear (Solberg, 1983). If our current disease indicators are valid, approximately two-thirds of the general population suffer from TM disorders. This figure obviously includes too many false-positive readings and illustrates that the application of a narrow set of examination criteria for functional correctness carries with it the danger of finding many people to be incorrectly diagnosed (Greene and Marbach, 1982). Despite this over-representation of disease, the false-negative situation is still possible. Only about one-fifth of radiographically documented cases with rheumatoid arthritis exhibit signs and symptoms at the time of examination (Ericsson and Lundberg, 1967; Ogus, 1975), and only 55 to 65% do so during the course of the disease (Ericsson and Lundberg, 1967; Ogus, 1975; Larheim *et al.,* 1982). Due to this poor performance of the presently accepted disease indicators, the prevalence of TM disorders as a disease in general, and in the aged in particular, is not known.

As far as identifiable subgroups of TM disorders are concerned, age is regarded as a predisposing factor in osteoarthrosis, but there is no evidence of any functionally important age-dependent alteration in the joint tissues to indicate that aging plays a primary etiologic role (Kopp and Carlsson, 1988). With the possible exception of early infancy, rheumatoid arthritis may commence at any age (Grahame, 1985). The onset of rheumatoid arthritis of the TMJ often occurs in individuals in their mid-thirties (Kopp and Carlsson, 1988), but despite that, it should not be regarded as an age-related disease. Ehrlich and colleagues (1970) suggested that rheumatoid arthritis follows a different path in those who show the first sign in old age. The female preponderance seen in younger rheumatoid subjects tends to disappear in the later decades of life (Grahame, 1985). No epidemiological data are available relative to the age-related incidence of acute, traumatic arthritis and internal derangement of the TMJ. However, it is assumed that these conditions are more frequently observed in the young. A frequent condition in the middle aged and elderly, described as an acute inflammatory synovial reaction (resulting from the physical presence of microcrystals within the synovial cavity), is known for primarily affecting joints other than the TMJ (Grahame and Scott, 1970; Resnick and Niwayama, 1988).

CONCLUSIONS

1. Pain, in general, is perceived differently by the aged. Limited evidence further suggests decreased sensitivity to cutaneous pricking and increased sensitivity to deep somatic pain.

2. Neuralgias, headaches due to cerebrovascular disease, cervical osteoarthritis and giant cell arteritis, carotidynia, and glossodynia are clearly more frequent in the aged. However, headaches, in general, are less frequent in the elderly.

3. Evidence strongly suggests an age-related decline of motor function in the masticatory system. The age-related functional deficit is not necessarily observed during habitual performance unless the system is compromised, for example, by drug-induced neuromuscular effects or masticatory dysfunction. If functional demands can no longer be met, coping strategies will be put into effect. Of particular concern are swallowing dysfunctions, with the possible disastrous consequence of laryngeal food spills.

4. A neglected dentition with loss of teeth is more prevalent in the aged. With respect to tooth loss, symptomatic subjects show a similar or less favorable dental status than asymptomatic subjects.

5. Psychophysiological factors are of importance in the etiology of TM disorders. Limited empirical evidence suggests differences in how the aged deal with or adapt to stress. Also, the extent to which frequently observed depressive preoccupations may affect pain tolerance in the aged and how this may relate to TM disorders is speculative at this time.

6. The extent of the problem of parafunctional oral habits in the aged is not known at this time.

7. At present, recognizing the limitation of the cross-sectional assessment of the age effect, epidemiological data regarding the frequency of commonly accepted disease descriptors do not suggest a strong age-related effect with respect to the prevalence or incidence of symptomatic subjects.

8. The prevalence of TM disorders in general, and in the aged in particular, is not known. However, empirical data do not suggest that age is a major risk factor.

9. With respect to identifiable subgroups of TM disorders, age may be regarded as a predisposing, rather than a primary etiologic factor in the osteoarthrosis of the TMJ. Rheumatoid arthritis of the TMJ should not be regarded as age-related. The age-associated incidence of acute mas-

ticatory muscle disorders, internal derangements and acute, traumatic arthritis of the TMJ is not known, however, empirical data suggest that these are more frequent in the young and middle aged.

REFERENCES

Agate, J. Common symptoms and complaints. In: *Clinical Geriatrics.* 3rd Ed. I. Rossman (Ed.), Lippincott, Philadelphia, 1986.

Agerberg, G. Maximal mandibular movements in young men and women. Sven. Tandlak. Tidskr. *67:*81-100, 1974*b*.

Agerberg, G. and G.E. Carlsson. Functional disorders of the masticatory system. II. Symptoms in relation to impaired mobility of the mandible as judged from investigation by questionnaire. Acta Odontol. Scand. *31:*335-347, 1973.

Agerberg, G. and G.E. Carlsson. Late results of treatment of functional disorders of the masticatory system. A follow-up by questionnaire. J. Oral Rehabil. *1:*309-316, 1974.

Agerberg, G. and G.E. Carlsson. Symptoms of functional disturbances of the masticatory system. A comparison of frequencies in a population sample and in a group of patients. Acta Odontol. Scand. *33:*183-190, 1975.

Aniansson, A. Muscle function in old age with special reference to muscle morphology, effect of training and capacity in activities of daily living. Doctoral dissertation, University of Göteborg, Göteborg, 1980.

Aniansson, A., G. Grimby, M. Hedberg and M. Krotkiewski. Muscle morphology, enzyme activity and muscle strength in elderly men and women. Clin. Physiol. *1:*73-86, 1981.

Aniansson, A., G. Grimby, M. Hedberg, A. Rungren and L. Sperling. Muscle function in old age. Scand. J. Rehabil. Med. *6:*43-49, 1978.

Argov, Z. and F.L. Mastaglia. Disorders of neuromuscular transmission caused by drugs. New Engl. J. Med. *301:*409-413, 1979.

Bates, J.F., G.D. Stafford and A. Harrison. Masticatory function—A review of the literature. II. Speed of movement of the mandible, rate of chewing and forces developed in chewing, 1975.

Baum, B.J. Aging and oral motor function. In: *Oral Motor Behavior. Impact on Oral Conditions and Dental Treatment.* P. Bryant, E. Gale and J. Rugh (Eds.), U.S.D.H.E.W., N.I.H. Publication No. 79-1845, Washington, D.C., 1979.

Behjou, S. and C.S. Stohler. Maximum mouth opening and orofacial pain. J. Dent. Res. *67(Special Issue)*:271, 1988.

Bell, W.E. Classification of TM disorders. In: *The President's Conference on the Examination, Diagnosis and Management of Temporomandibular Disorders.* D. Laskin *et al.*, (Eds.), American Dental Association, Chicago, 1983.

Bell, W.E. *Orofacial Pains. Classification, Diagnosis and Management.* 3rd Ed. YearBook Medical Publishers, Chicago, 1985.

Blazer, D. and C.D. Williams. Epidemiology of dysphoria and depression in an elderly population. Am. J. Psychiatry *137:*439-444, 1980.

Bosma, J.F. Sensorimotor examination of the mouth and pharynx. Front. Oral Physiol. *2:*78-107, 1976.

Bosman, A. *Hinge Axis Determination of the Mandible.* Stagleu & Tholen, Leiden, 1974.

Burke, R.E., D.N. Levin, P. Tsairis and F.E. Zajac. Physiological types and histochemical profiles in motor units of the cat gastrocnemius. J. Physiol. *234:*723-748, 1973.

Chapman, W.P. and C.M. Jones. Variation in cutaneous and visceral pain sensitivity in normal subjects. J. Clin. Invest. *23:*81-91, 1944.

Cheshire, C.M. and W.J.K. Cumming. The musculoskeletal system—Skeletal muscle. In: *Textbook of Geriatric Medicine and Gerontology.* 3rd Ed., J.C. Brocklehurst (Ed.), Churchill Livinstone, Edinburgh, 1985.

Clarkson, P.M., W. Kroll and A.M. Melchionda. Age, isometric strength, rate of tension development and fibre type composition. J. Gerontol. *36:*648-653, 1981.

Cunningham, D.A., P.A. Rechnitzer, M.E. Peare and A.P. Donner. Determinants of self-selected walking pace across 19 to 66. J. Gerontol. *37:*560-564, 1982.

DeBoever, J.A. and P.A. Adriaens. Occlusal relationship in patients with pain-dysfunction symptoms in the temporomandibular joints. J. Oral Rehabil. *10:*1-7, 1983.

Egermark-Eriksson, I. Malocclusion and some functional recordings of the masticatory system in Swedish school children. Swed. Dent. J. *6:*9-20, 1982.

Egermark-Eriksson, I., B. Ingervall and G.E. Carlsson. The dependence of mandibular dysfunction in children on functional and morphologic malocclusion. Am. J. Orthod. *83:*187-194, 1983.

Ehrlich, G.E., W.A. Katz and S.H. Cohen. Rheumatoid arthritis in the elderly. Geriatrics *2:*103-113, 1970.

Ericsson, S. and M. Lundberg. Alterations in the temporomandibular joint at various stages of rheumatoid arthritis. Acta Rheum. Scand. *13:*257-274, 1967.

Eversole, L.R. *Clinical Outline of Oral Pathology. Diagnosis and Treatment.* Lea and Febiger, Philadelphia, 1978.

Forssell, H. Mandibular dysfunction and headache. Proc. Finn. Dent. Soc. *81(Suppl. 2)*, 1985.

Franks, A.S.T. The dental health of patients presenting with temporomandibular joint dysfunction. Brit. J. Oral Surg. *5:*157-166, 1968.

Franks, A.S.T. and B. Hedegard. *Geriatric Dentistry.* Blackwell Scientific Publications, Oxford, 1973.

Gardner, D.I. and P. O'Connor. The musculoskeletal system—Aging of articular cartilage. In: *Textbook of Geriatric Medicine and Gerontology.* 3rd Ed., J.C. Brocklehurst (Ed.), Churchill Livingstone, Edinburgh, 1985.

Geering, A.H. Occlusal interferences and functional disturbances of the masticatory system. J. Clin. Periodontol. *1:*112-119, 1974.

Gianturco, D.T. and E.W. Busse. Psychiatric problems encountered during a long-term study of normal ageing volunteers. In: *Studies in Geriatric Psychiatry.* A.D. Isaac and F. Post (Eds.), Wiley, Chichester, 1978.

Glaros, A.G. Incidence of diurnal and nocturnal bruxism. J. Prosthet. Dent. *45:*545-549, 1981.

Grahame, R. The musculoskeletal system—Disease of the joints. In: *Textbook of Geriatric Medicine and Gerontology.* 3rd Ed., J.C. Brocklehurst (Ed.), Churchill Livingstone, Edinburgh, 1985.

Grahame, R. and J.T. Scott. Clinical survey of 354 patients with gout. Ann. Rheum. Dis. *29:*461-468, 1970.

Greene, C.S. and J.J. Marbach. Epidemiological studies of mandibular dysfunction: A critical review. J. Prosthet. Dent. *48:*184-190, 1982.

Grimby, G., B. Danneskijold-Samsoe, K. Hvid and B. Saltin. Morphology and enzymatic capacity in arm and leg muscles in 78-81 year old men and women. Acta Physiol. Scand. *115:*125-134, 1982.

Gurland, B.J., L. Dean, P. Cross and R. Golden. The epidemiology of depression and dementia in the elderly: The use of multiple indicators of these conditions. In: *Psychopathology in the Aged.* J.O. Cole and J.E. Barrett (Eds.), Raven Press, New York, 1980.

Gutmann, E. Muscle. In: *The Biology of Aging.* C.E. Finch and L. Hayflick (Eds.), Van Nostrand Reinhold, New York, 1977.

Hall, D.A. *The Biomedical Basis of Gerontology.* Wright, Bristol, 1984.

Hammerstadt, J.P. Headache and facial pain. In: *Geriatric Medicine.* Vol. I, C.K. Cassel and J.R. Walsh (Eds.), Springer, New York, 1985.

Hansson, T. and M. Nilner. A study of the occurrence of symptoms of diseases of the temporomandibular joint masticatory musculature and related structures. J. Oral Rehabil. *2:*313-324, 1975.

Haraldsson, T., U. Karlsson and G.E. Carlsson. Bite force and oral function in complete denture wearers. J. Oral Rehabil. *6:*41-48, 1979.

Harkins, S.W. and M.H. Warner. Age and pain. In: *Annual Review of Gerodontology and Geriatrics.* Vol. 1, S. Eisendorfer (Ed.), Springer, New York, 1980.

Hartmann, E. Alcohol and bruxism. N. Engl. J. Med. *301:*333-334, 1979.

Helkimo, M. Studies on the function and dysfunction of the masticatory system. Proc. Finn. Dent. Soc. *70:*37-49, 1974*a*.

Helkimo, M. Studies on function and dysfunction of the masticatory system. II. Index for anamnestic and clinical dysfunction and occlusal state. Swed. Dent. J. *67:*101-121, 1974*b*.

Helkimo, M. Studies on function and dysfunction of the masticatory system. III. Analyses of anamnestic and clinical recordings of dysfunction with the aid of indices. Swed. Dent. J. *67:*165-181, 1974*c*.

Heloe, B. and L.A. Heloe. Frequency and distribution of myofascial pain-dysfunction syndrome in a population of 25-year olds. Comm. Dent. Oral Epidemiol. *7:*357-360, 1979.

Heloe, L.A. Comparison of dental health data obtained from questionnaires, interviews and clinical examination. Scand. J. Dent. Res. *80:*495-499, 1972.

Heyck, H. *Headache and Facial Pain. Differential Diagnosis, Pathogenesis and Treatment.* Thieme, Stuttgart, 1981.

Hodgson, S.P. and D.J. Jolley. Psychiatry of the elderly. In: *Principles and Practice of Geriatric Medicine.* M.S.J. Pathy (Ed.), Wiley, Chichester, 1985.

Hudgson, P. Adverse drug reactions in the neuromuscular apparatus. Adv. Drug React. Acute Pois. Rev. *1:*35-64, 1982.

Ingervall, B., B. Mohlin and B. Thilander. Prevalence of symptoms of functional disturbances of the masticatory system in Swedish men. J. Oral Rehabil. *7:*185-197, 1980.

Kamen, S. Tardive dyskinesia, a significant syndrome for geriatric dentistry. Oral Surg., Oral Med., Oral Path. *39:*52-57, 1975.

Kline, N.S. On the rarity of irreversible oral dyskinesia following phenothiazines. Am. J. Psychiatry *124:*48-54, 1968.

Kolodny, A.L. and A.R. Klipper. Bone and joint diseases in the elderly. Hosp. Pract. *11:*91-101, 1976.

Kopp, S. and G.E. Carlsson. The temporomandibular joint: Problems related to occlusal function. In: *A Textbook of Occlusion.* N.D. Mohl, G.A. Zarb, G.E. Carlsson, and J.D. Rugh (Eds.), Quintessence, Chicago, 1988.

Kudrow, L. *Cluster Headache, Mechanisms and Management.* Oxford University Press, Oxford, 1980.

Lance, J.W., D.A. Curran and M. Anthony. Investigations into the mechanism and treatment of chronic headache. Med. J. Aust. *2:*909-914, 1965.

Larheim, T.A., H.M. Hoyeraal, A.E. Stabrun, and H.R. Haanees. The temporomandibular joint in juvenile rheumatoid arthritis. Scand. J. Rheumatol. *11:*5-12, 1982.

Larsson, L., B. Sjodin and J. Karlsson. Histochemical and biomechanical changes in human skeletal muscle with age in sedentary males aged 22-65 years. Acta Physiol. Scand. *103:*31-39, 1978.

Larsson, L. Morphological and functional characteristics of aging skeletal muscle in man. Acta Physiol. Scand. *103(Suppl. 457), 1978.*

Lindqvist, B. Bruxism in children. Odontol. Revy *22:*413-423, 1971.

Lindqvist, B. Bruxism and emotional disturbance. Odontol. Revy *23:*231-242, 1972.

Lindqvist, B. and J. Heijbel. Bruxism in children with brain damage. Acta Odontol. Scand. *32:*313-319, 1974.

Lysell, L. Epidemiologisk-rontgendiagnostik undersoking av tander, kakar och kakleder hos 67-ar-ingar i dalby. Doctoral dissertation, University of Malmö, Malmö, 1977.

MacLennan, W.J., M.R.P. Hall, J.I. Timothy and M. Robinson. Is weakness in old age due to muscle wasting? Age and Ageing *9:*188-192, 1980.

Magnusson, T. and G.E. Carlsson. A 2 1/2 year follow-up of changes in headache and mandibular dysfunction after stomatognathic treatment. J. Prosthet. Dent. *49:*398-402, 1983.

Magnusson, T. *Mandibular Dysfunction and Recurrent Headache.* Doctoral dissertation, University of Göteborg, Göteborg, 1981.

Makila, E. Frequency of mandibular dysfunction symptoms in institutionalized elderly people. Gerontology *25:*238-243, 1979.

Maruyama, T., S. Miyauchi and E. Umekoji. Analysis of the mandibular relationship of TMJ dysfunction patients using the Mandibular Kinesiograph. J. Oral Rehabil. *9:*217-223, 1982.

Maxwell, L.C., D.S. Carlson, J.A. McNamara and J.A. Faulkner. Histochemical characteristics of the masseter and temporalis muscles of the rhesus monkey *(Macaca mulatta).* Anat. Rec. *193:*389-403, 1979.

McCarter, R. Effects of age on the contraction of mammalian skeletal muscle. In: *Aging in Muscles.* G. Kaldor and W.J. Battista (Eds.), Raven Press, New York, 1978.

Meklas, J.F. Bruxism. Diagnosis and treatment. J. Acad. Gen. Dent. *19:*31-36, 1971.

Mohl, N.D. The temporomandibular joint. In: *A Textbook of Occlusion.* N.D. Mohl, G.A. Zarb, G.E. Carlsson and J.D. Rugh (Eds.), Quintessence, Chicago, 1988.

Molin, C., G. Edman and D. Schalling. Psychological studies of patients with mandibular pain dysfunction syndrome. M.D.S. II: Tolerance for experimentally induced pain. Swed. Dent. J. *66:*15-23, 1973.

Molin, C., G.E. Carlsson, B. Friling and B. Hedegard. Frequency of symptoms of mandibular dysfunction in young Swedish men. J. Oral Rehabil. *3:*9-18, 1976.

Mongini, F. Remodelling of the mandibular condyle in the adult and its relationship to the condition of the dental arches. Acta Anat. *82:*437-453, 1972.

Mumford, J.M. Pain perception in man on electrically stimulating the teeth. In: *Pain.* A. Soulairac, J. Cahn and J. Charpentier (Eds.), Academic Press, London, 1968.

Nevakari, K. "Elapsio praearticularis" of the temporomandibular joint. A pantographic study of the so-called physiologic subluxation. Acta Odontol. Scand. *18:*123-170, 1960.

Newland, C.A., L.S. Illis, P.K. Robinson, B.G. Batchelor and W.E. Waters. A survey of headache in an English city. Res. Clin. Stud. Headache *5:*1-20, 1978.

Oberg, T., G.E. Carlsson and C.M. Fajers. The temporomandibular joint: A morphological study on a human autopsy material. Acta Odontol. Scand. *29:*349-384, 1971.

Ogura, T., T. Morinushi, H. Ohno *et al.* An epidemiological study of TMJ dysfunction syndrome in adolescents. J. Pedodont. *10:*22-35, 1985.

Ogus, H. Rheumatoid arthritis of the temporomandibular joint. Brit. J. Oral Surg. *12:*275-284, 1975.

Osterberg, T. and G.E. Carlsson. Symptoms and signs of mandibular dysfunction in 70-year-old men and women in Gothenburg, Sweden. Comm. Dent. Oral Epidemiol. *7:*315-321, 1979.

Posselt, U. Studies in the mobility of the human mandible. Acta Odontol. Scand. *10(Suppl):*10, 1952.

Post, F. The central nervous system—The emotional disorders. In: *Textbook of Geriatric Medicine and Gerontology.* 3rd Ed., J.C. Brocklehurst (Ed.), Churchill Livingstone, Edinburgh, 1985.

Procacci, P., G. Bozza, G. Buzzelli and M. Della-Corte. The cutaneous pricking pain threshold in old age. In: *Pain. Clinical and Experimental Perspectives.* M. Weisenberg (Ed.), C.V. Mosby Co., St. Louis, 1985.

Reding, G.R., W.C. Rubright and S.O. Zimmerman. Incidence of bruxism. J. Dent. Res. *45:*1198-1204, 1966.

Resnick, D. and G. Niwayama. Gouty arthritis. In: *Diagnosis of Bone and Joint Disorders.* 2nd Ed., D. Resnick and G. Niwayama (Eds.), W.B. Saunders, Philadelphia, 1988.

Richmond, G.H., J.D. Rugh, R. Dolfi and R.R Lemke. Masticatory conditions of the institutionalized mentally retarded. J. Dent. Res. *60(Special Issue):*425, 1981.

Rieder, C.E. Comparison of the efficacy of a questionnaire, oral history and clinical examination in detecting signs and symptoms of occlusal and temporomandibular joint dysfunction. J. Prosthet. Dent. *38:*433-440, 1977.

Ringqvist, M. Histochemical fiber types and fiber sizes in human masticatory muscles. Scand. J. Dent. Res. *79:*366-368, 1971.

Ringqvist, M. Histochemical enzyme profiles of fibres in human masseter muscles with special regard to fibres with intermediate myofibrillar ATPase reaction. J. Neurol. Sci. *18:*133-141, 1973.

Rugh, J.D. Psychological components of pain. Dent. Clin. N. Am. *31(4):*579-594, 1987.

Rugh, J.D. and J. Harlan. Nocturnal bruxism and temporomandibular disorders. In: *Advances in Neurology. Facial Dyskinesias.* Vol. 49, J. Jankovic and E. Tolosa (Eds.), Raven Press, New York, 1988.

Schluderman, E. and J.P. Zubeck. Effect of age on pain sensitivity. Percept. Mot. Skills *14:*295-301, 1952.

Seligman, D.A., A.G. Pullinger and W.K. Solberg. The prevalence of dental attrition and its association with factors of age, gender, occlusion, and TMJ symptomatology. J. Dent. Res. *67:*1323-1333, 1988.

Sessle, B.J. Neurophysiology of orofacial pain. Dent. Clin. N. Am. *31(4):* 595-613, 1987*a*.

Sessle, B.J. The neurobiology of facial and dental pain. J. Dent. Res. *66:*962-981, 1987*b*.

Sherman, E.D. and E. Robillard. Sensitivity to pain in relationship to age. In: *Age with a Future: Proceedings of the 6th International Congress of Gerontology.* P.F. Hansen (Ed.), Davis, Philadelphia, 1964.

Shikata, H., N. Utsumi and D. Fujimoto. Collagen in aging bones of the jaw. Front. Oral Physiol. *6:*85-95, 1987.

Shock, N.W. Longitudinal studies of aging in humans. In: *Handbook of the Biology of Aging.* 2nd Ed., C.E. Finch and E.L. Schneider (Ed.), Van Nostrand Reinhold, New York, 1985.

Solberg, W.K., M.W. Woo and J.B. Houston. Prevalence of mandibular dysfunction in young adults. J. Am. Dent. Assoc. *98:*25-34, 1979.

Solberg, W.K. Epidemiology, incidence and prevalence of temporomandibular disorders: A review. In: *The President's Conference on the Examination, Diagnosis and Management of Temporomandibular Disorders.* D. Laskin *et al.* (Eds.), American Dental Association, Chicago, 1983.

Stenback, A., M. Kumperlainen and M.L. Vauhkonen. A field study of old age depression. In: *Recent Advances in Gerontology.* H. Orima *et al.* (Eds), Int. Congress Series (n. 469), Excerpta Medica, Amsterdam, 1979.

Storey, A.T. Neurophysiological aspects of TM disorders. In: *The President's Conference on the Examination, Diagnosis and Management of Temporomandibular Disorders.* D. Laskin *et al.,* (Eds.), American Dental Association, Chicago, 1983.

Strehler, B.L. Aging and the human brain. In: *Neurobiology of Aging.* R.D. Terry and S. Gershon (Eds.), Raven Press, New York, 1976.

Swanljung, O. and T. Rantanen. Functional disorders of the masticatory system in southwest Finland. Comm. Dent. Oral Epidemiol. *7:*177-182, 1979.

Tallgren, A. Electromyographic study of the behavior of certain facial and jaw muscles in long-term complete denture wearers. Odontol. Tidskr. *71:*425-444, 1963.

Thompson, R.H., A.M. Geiger, B.H. Wasserman and T. Turgeon. Relationship of occlusion and peridontal disease. Part III. Relation of periodontal status to general background characteristics. J. Periodontol. *43:*540-546, 1972.

Thomson, H. Mandibular dysfunction syndrome. Brit. Dent. J. *130:*187-193, 1971.

Tobin, S.S. Psychological adaptation to stress by the elderly. In: *Homeostatic Function and Aging.* B.B. Davis and W.G. Wood (Eds.), Raven Press, New York, 1985.

Travell, J. Temporomandibular joint pain referred from muscles of the head and neck. J. Prosthet. Dent. *10:*745-763, 1960.

Vanderspek, A.F.L., W.B. Fang, J.A. Ashton-Miller, C.S. Stohler, D.S. Carlson and M.A. Schork. Increased masticatory muscle stiffness during limb muscle flaccidity associated with succinylcholine administration. Anesthesiology *69:*11-16, 1988.

Waters, W.E. The Pontypridd headache survey. Headache *14:*81-90, 1974.

Watkin, D.M. The physiology of aging. Am. J. Clin. Nutr. *36:*750, 1982.

Weissman, M.M., J.K. Myers and W.D. Thompson. Affective disorders in an urban U.S. community. Arch. Gen. Psychiatr. *38:*417-421, 1981.

Welford, A.T. Principles of motor control and their application to dental problems. In: *Oral Motor Behavior: Impact on Oral Conditions and Dental Treatment.* P. Bryant, E. Gale and J. Rugh (Eds.), U.S.D.H.E.W., N.I.H. Publication No. 79-1845, Washington, D.C., 1979.

Welford, A.T. Changes of performance with age. An overview. In: *Aging and Human Performance.* N. Charness (Ed.), Wiley, Chichester, 1985.

Wigdorowicz-Makowerowa, N., C. Grodzki, H. Panek, T. Maslanka, K. Plonka and A. Palacha. Epidemiologic studies on prevalence and etiology of functional disturbances of the masticatory system. J. Prosthet. Dent. *41:*76-82, 1979.

Woodrow, K.M., G.D. Friedman, A.B. Siegelaub *et al.* Differences according to age, sex and race. Psychosom. Med. *34:*548-556, 1972.

Zarb, G.A. Oral motor behaviors and oral prostheses. In: *Oral Motor Behavior: Impact on Oral Conditions and Dental Treatment.* P. Bryant, E. Gale and J. Rugh (Eds.), U.S.D.H.E.W., N.I.H. Publication No. 79-1845, Washington, D.C., 1979.

Zarb, G.A. and N.D. Mohl. Occlusion and temporomandibular disorders: A prologue. In: *A Textbook of Occlusion.* N.D. Mohl, G.A. Zarb, G.E. Carlsson and J.D. Rugh (Eds.), Quintessence, Chicago, 1988.

Zarb, G.A. and G.W. Thompson. The treatment of patients with temporomandibular joint pain dysfunction syndrome. J. Can. Dent. Assoc. *41:*410-417, 1975.

ORTHODONTICS IN AN AGING SOCIETY: AN OVERVIEW

William R. Proffit

In developing an overview of orthodontics in an aging society, it is important to consider the subject from three perspectives: (1) that of society; (2) that of orthodontists, or more broadly, those who deliver health care; and (3), most importantly, that of the older patients who now are seeking orthodontic treatment.

THE AGING SOCIETY

Although it is correct to characterize our society as an aging one, it is more accurate to describe society as having a middle-aged bulge (Achenbaum, 1989; Halter, 1989). There are now more people in the group between 30 and 60 years of age than ever before, and in absolute numbers this is the most rapidly growing part of the population. If percentages are used, the over-80 age group is the fastest growing part of the population, but in absolute numbers the vast majority of the population will continue to be younger than that. It is those in the middle age group, individuals who are older than those who have traditionally sought orthodontic treatment but who are not really aged, who will become important for orthodontists in the future.

Although the absolute number of children, and not just the proportion of children in the population, is decreasing, this may not mean that orthodontists will have fewer child patients. As we come to have relatively fewer children in our society, we may well value them more and be more likely to seek treatment for them. Although it seems strange to think of children that way, the notion that scarcity of an entity or object tends to increase its perceived value applies to them as well. There is nothing novel in the observation that a child in a family of one or two children gets more individual attention than a child in a large family. As couples wait until they have reached an older age to have children, compared to couples in previous years, they tend to become concerned parents who are more likely to seek orthodontic treatment for their child than parents in the past. Interestingly enough, these older parents also seem to be more likely to take their child to an orthodontist for consultation at age six or seven, instead of waiting until an orthodontic problem has become obvious, often not until the age of eleven or twelve. The age range for orthodontic treatment, in short, is likely to be extended in both directions, with an assist from these older parents.

An increased focus on children is much easier for affluent individuals with small families. While this description characterizes a considerable proportion of our society, there are many families to which it does not apply. In the future, not only will there be fewer children, but more of them will be from minority groups. The plight of disadvantaged children who need treatment but are unable to receive it because of social and economic constraints must not be ignored. If, as seems likely, our society develops a family health care policy, dental and orthodontic needs should be included.

ORTHODONTIC PRACTICE IN THE AGING SOCIETY

Another impending demographic change of importance for orthodontists, in addition to the change in the age mix in the population of patients, is a change in the age and sex mix within the orthodontic community itself. The era of rapid expansion in the number of orthodontists has ended, and the inevitable result will be a gradual increase in the average age of practitioners. Until recently, very few women were trained as orthodontic specialists, but that has changed dramatically. At present, approximately one-third of those in training are female. The younger segment of the professional group, therefore, will have a very different sex ratio than previously, which will undoubtedly affect the pattern of practice.

The greatest impact on orthodontists, however, is likely to result from a decline in the number of young women who are available as clinical assistants. The traditional practice staffed with a large number of energetic young women is simply not going to be possible in the future. Orthodontic practices will have to employ older individuals as clinical assistants, with all that implies in working styles and conditions. A young person who expects to work in a practice for only a few years will accept lower wages, fewer fringe benefits and poorer working conditions than a long-term employee who sees assisting as a career. However, there will be an integral role for career-oriented people in staffing orthodontic practices in the future.

THE OLDER ORTHODONTIC PATIENT

Patients seek orthodontic treatment at older ages for two major reasons which themselves are correlated with age. At present, the majority of adult orthodontic patients are in the 25 to 40 age range. At this age, adults who desire orthodontic treatment usually are seeking a general improvement, not only in dental health and esthetics but also in their life situation. A typical situation might be the 32-year-old assistant professor who has always wanted to have his teeth straightened. Now he can afford it. Besides, he estimates that the chances of tenure and an eventual department chairmanship might be better with teeth that no longer detract from his appearance. The number of people who seek orthodontic treatment for these reasons falls off sharply above age 40.

The second major group of adults, the group who are becoming increasingly important as the population ages, are those who seek orthodontics because they have specific health care needs for which orthodontic treatment is important. They seek orthodontic consultation because the periodontist told them that they may lose their teeth unless something is done, or the prosthodontist said that without orthodontics, there is no way to make a bridge. These are individuals whose treatment Melsen discusses in this volume. They tend to be in the 40 to 60 age range, although they can be younger or older. This is the group that will provide the greatest increase in the numbers of adult orthodontic patients in the future, simply because of the population bulge.

LIMITATIONS OF ORTHODONTIC TREATMENT IN ADULTS

Envelope of Discrepancy

There are some inherent limitations in the potential of orthodontic treatment for adults in any age group, compared to adolescents and children. One important limitation relates to what James Ackerman and I have called the "envelope of discrepancy" which is illustrated in Figure 1 and shows the maximum size of a discrepancy that can be corrected by (1) tooth movement alone (the inner circle); (2) tooth movement coupled with growth modification (the middle circle); and (3) orthognathic surgery (the outer circle). The concept is more important than the precise numbers. There may be some debate as to whether a lower incisor can be advanced more or less than the 5 mm suggested by the model, but there is no doubt that a greater reduction in overjet can be achieved

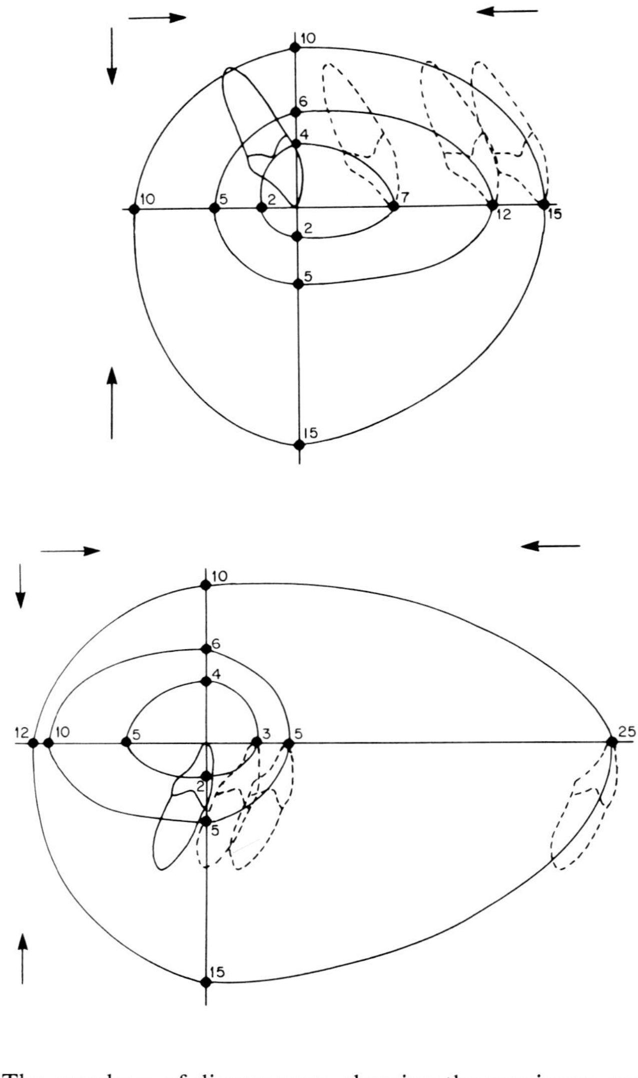

Figure 1. The envelope of discrepancy, showing the maximum correction of an occlusal discrepancy that can be expected from tooth movement alone (the inner circle), tooth movement combined with growth modification (the middle circle), and orthognathic surgery (the outer circle) for the upper jaw (top) and lower jaw (bottom). Because the inner circle is the only possibility for orthodontic treatment of adults, surgery is required for satisfactory correction of some problems that could have been treated orthodontically at an earlier age. (Redrawn from Proffit and Ackerman, 1985.)

through a combination of growth modification and orthodontic tooth movement than through orthodontic tooth movement alone. Growth modification is possible, of course, only in individuals who have a significant amount of growth remaining. It is for this reason that the potential change that can be produced through orthodontic treatment is significantly less for adults than for children. This is also the reason that some problems which could be solved in a child by orthodontic treatment that includes growth modification would require orthognathic surgery for satisfactory correction if encountered in an adult.

Systemic and Local Factors

A number of other systemic and local factors can produce limitations on orthodontic treatment possibilities for adults. For example, there is a remarkable increase in diabetes in patients above age 45 (Halter, 1989). Diabetes is not a trivial matter in any circumstances, but it is particularly serious for a patient who is undergoing orthodontic treatment, because of the rapid and progressive periodontal bone loss that can occur in diabetic patients. What the host of potential systemic and local factors mean, as Dr. Melsen points out in her article in this volume, is that in order to treat adults successfully, it is necessary to work with other care providers in order to meet the patient's needs. For patients with diabetes, arthritis, or other health problems, it becomes increasingly important to coordinate orthodontic treatment with other health care as the patient grows older.

Patient Compliance

Another difference between adults and children with regard to orthodontics is the degree of emotional involvement with the treatment. Many children react to orthodontic treatment in exactly the same way they react to school, church, dancing lessons, summer camp, and a host of other required activities: they more or less passively go along with what their parents want, without making a real commitment to it themselves. An adult does not choose to have orthodontic treatment if he or she is indifferent to the whole idea. The good news about this fact is that it is not hard to get most adults to brush their teeth, wear their rubber bands and keep their appointments. The bad news is that treatment for an adult is likely to take more of the orthodontist's time, because the orthodontist will have no choice but to meet the adult patient's need for feedback on treatment progress. It is important to meet the adult's emotional as well as physical needs, and that takes time.

TMJ Problems

The prevalence of temporomandibular joint problems as a function of age is interesting. As Dr. Stohler points out in his paper in this volume, myofascial pain-dysfunction and other TMJ problems are not particularly a problem of an aging population. There is a peak incidence of TMJ problems in individuals who are in their twenties and thirties; after that, they stabilize or even decline. TMJ problems are concentrated in the younger adult group rather than the older one. Nevertheless, these problems do have to be treated in some adult patients. It is fortunate that rational and professional methods now seem to be replacing the largely empirical and frequently irrational approaches to these problems used in recent years.

Orthodontic Mechanotherapy

The orthodontic mechanotherapy needed to treat adults is often more complex than that required in treatment of children. One major reason is that it is necessary to intrude teeth in order to correct vertical problems in adults. That, in turn, requires the use of segmented arch rather than continuous arch mechanics. The examples presented by Dr. Melsen in this volume are excellent illustrations of the application of the segmented arch technique to the treatment of adults with periodontal problems. The continuous arch approach that most orthodontists use most of the time is entirely satisfactory for treatment of the majority of children and some adults. It is fair to say, however, that an orthodontist who cannot handle segmented arch mechanics will be in increasing trouble as the number of adult patients in his or her practice increases, particularly as the older patients with specific health needs replace the younger ones who are seeking general improvement.

Surgical Orthodontics

Whether an adult needs combined surgical and orthodontic treatment rather than orthodontics alone is determined by two factors: the severity of the malocclusion, and the benefits to be gained from correcting it. The envelope of discrepancy (Fig. 1) illustrates reasonably well the limitations of orthodontic relative to surgical treatment, but of course it does not imply that orthognathic surgery is required for everyone who has a malocclusion too severe to be corrected through orthodontics; the degree of improvement the treatment is considered likely to provide must determine that. The borderline patient, whose malocclusion is too severe to correct orthodontically without exceeding the bounds of reasonable compromise and yet not so obviously bad that the patient would readily accept surgery, is the problem. The best way to choose between two treatment approaches is to consider their relative benefits and the risks and cost of each. If extensive orthodontic treatment is considered likely to produce little benefit in a given case, it would be very difficult to justify this over an admittedly riskier and costlier surgical procedure that is considered likely to produce considerable benefit. Approaching cost-benefit and risk-benefit openly and explicitly with the patient can help a great deal.

Adjunctive Orthodontics

Older patients often require different orthodontic treatment in another sense, because what they need often is adjunctive rather than comprehensive orthodontics. In any treatment, the goal should be to maximize benefit for that individual. Maximum benefit for a 50-year-old patient with periodontal disease may mean aligning the incisors so that periodontal splinting can be carried out, while leaving a posterior crossbite uncorrected. What would be entirely appropriate for a 55-year-old may be less appropriate for a 15-year-old, and vice versa.

Whatever the goals of treatment are, they should be precisely outlined at the beginning, and the treatment should be aimed at reaching that goal. A compromise aimed at maximizing benefit to the patient by no means is inferior orthodontics. By the same token, treatment that does not meet its goals should not be dignified by the after-the-fact title of limited adjunctive treatment.

Growth in the Adult

A final point of considerable interest in clinical orthodontics is the meaning of Dr. Behrents' material on continued growth of the jaws in adults, discussed in his paper in this volume. It is fascinating to learn that adults continue to grow. On the other hand, it is important to look at the growth quantitatively. The amount of change that will occur due to growth in individuals after the age of 30 is large enough to detect, but not large enough to cause the kind of post-treatment change that is normal in a 12-year-old. Relapse due to growth will be rare in adult patients. Perhaps the most valuable part of Dr. Behrents' work is its demonstration that we have often been too pessimistic about the amount of growth that can occur in late adolescence. There is more growth potential after puberty than many of us had thought.

SUMMARY

In summary, the practice of orthodontics in an aging society will indeed be conducted differently than in the typical practice of the past. The societal emphasis, the nature of orthodontic practice, and the age mix of the patients will change. There is every reason to believe, however, that orthodontics will continue to be a prominent and valued part of dental practice.

REFERENCES

Achenbaum, W.A. The aging society. In: *Orthodontics in an Aging Society.* D.S. Carlson (Ed.), Monograph 22, Craniofacial Growth Series, Center for Human Growth and Development, The University of Michigan, Ann Arbor, 1989.

Behrents, R.G. The consequences of adult craniofacial growth. In: *Orthodontics in an Aging Society.* D.S. Carlson (Ed.), Monograph 22, Craniofacial Growth Series, Center for Human Growth and Development, The University of Michigan, Ann Arbor, 1989.

Halter, J.B. Clinical implications of the aging process. In: *Orthodontics in an Aging Society.* D.S. Carlson (Ed.), Monograph 22, Craniofacial Growth Series, Center for Human Growth and Development, The University of Michigan, Ann Arbor, 1989.

Melsen, B. Orthodontic treatment of the degenerated dentition. In: *Orthodontics in an Aging Society.* D.S. Carlson (Ed.), Monograph 22, Craniofacial Growth Series, Center for Human Growth and Development, The University of Michigan, Ann Arbor, 1989.

Proffit, W.R. and J. Ackerman. Diagnosis and treatment planning in orthodontics. In: *Orthodontics: Current Concepts and Techniques.* T.M. Graber and B.F. Swain (Eds.), C.V. Mosby Co., St. Louis, 1985.

Stohler, C.S. Temporomandibular disorders in the aged. In: *Orthodontics in an Aging Society.* D.S. Carlson (Ed.), Monograph 22, Craniofacial Growth Series, Center for Human Growth and Development, The University of Michigan, Ann Arbor, 1989.

THE TIMING OF SECONDARY SEX CHARACTERISTICS AND THEIR RELATIONSHIP TO THE PUBERTAL MAXIMUM OF GROWTH IN BOYS

Urban Hägg
Johan Karlberg
John Taranger

It has been shown by Björk (1972) that there is a close temporal association between maximum pubertal growth in facial dimensions and standing height. This association led Björk to recommend the use of individual velocity curves of standing height as an indirect tool to estimate the period of greatest rate of facial growth for use in orthodontic treatment planning. It has recently been shown (Hägg *et al.,* 1987; Hägg and Pancherz, 1988) that the greatest mandibular growth occurred in patients treated either in the annual interval during which peak height velocity occurred or in the following year. Accordingly, in treatment involving orthopedic appliances during a relatively short period of time (6-12 months), the period during which the pubertal maximum of standing height occurs, or just after it, may be a better time to affect growth than the beginning of the pubertal growth spurt or the late prepubertal period of growth of standing height, when the mandibular growth rate is low (Hägg *et al.,* 1987; Hägg and Pancherz, 1988).

The pubertal maximum in standing height occurs, on the average, at about 14 years of age. According to Björk (1972), the pubertal maximum in facial dimensions occurs simultaneously with that of standing height, or during the following year. The individual variation in the occurrence of the pubertal maximum is about six years, i.e., from 11.5 to 17.5 years (Hägg and Taranger, 1982). Accordingly, chronological age is not a good indicator of physical maturity.

Longitudinal records of standing height can be used to assess an individual's position on the facial growth curve (Björk, 1972). Velocity curves of standing height have been used in clinical studies of Herbst patients (Pancherz and Hägg, 1985; Hägg *et al.,* 1987; Hägg and

Pancherz, 1988). Distance curves of standing height (Karlberg, 1987) have been used in a clinical study involving patients treated with a modified activator appliance (Malmgren *et al.*, 1987), and in a study comparing the effect of the Herbst appliance and a modified activator appliance (Pancherz *et al.*, 1988). Such approaches require reliable serial data of height measurements.

In longitudinal and cross-sectional evaluation of an individual's somatic maturity one can use, for instance, assessments of hand-wrist radiographs and secondary sex characteristics as maturity indicators. The relationships between the stage of skeletal maturity and the increase of mandibular length in patients who had Class II malocclusions and who were treated with the Herbst appliance have been reported previously (Hägg *et al.*, 1987; Hägg and Pancherz, 1988). Some colleagues believe that the use of radiographic techniques for determining skeletal development, particularly in rapidly growing individuals, is of questionable value (e.g., George, 1987). Although direct questioning of patients regarding their own development in terms of secondary sex characteristics may not be feasible, it may in some cases be possible to obtain this information from the patient's physician.

The previous longitudinal studies on secondary sex characteristics and their relation to pubertal maximum growth in boys (e.g., Marshall and Tanner, 1970; Largo and Prader, 1983) have examined only a limited number of parameters. The aims of this study were to determine the timing of the secondary sex characteristics in a representative prospective sample of Swedish boys, and to describe the relation in time between these pubertal events and the pubertal maximum of growth.

SUBJECTS

Data has been collected from a random sample of 122 Swedish boys who were followed from birth to 25 years of age for a prospective longitudinal study (Karlberg *et al.*, 1976; Hägg, 1980). During the 9 to 21 years age period covered in this paper, annual registration of 8 signs of the development of the secondary sex characteristics were made in boys to 18 years of age, and follow-up registrations were made at 21 and 25 years. At the age of 18 years, 75% of the original boys were still participating in the study. Between 9 and 18 years of age, 22 out of 112 boys left the study.

METHODS OF REGISTRATION

Two examiners performed over 90% of the registrations in this study (Karlberg *et al.*, 1976). Height was measured with the stretching-up technique (Weiner and Lourie, 1969) and recorded in millimeters. During the period between 10 to 18 years of age, height was measured every three months.

The ratings of the secondary sex characteristics were made by visual inspection at the clinical examination of the children without knowledge of previous ratings. The genital maturity of boys was always assessed visually prior to estimation of testicular volume by means of an orchidometer (Prader, 1966; Marshall and Tanner, 1986). The definitions of stages of pubertal development used (Tanner, 1962; Prader, 1966; Marshall and Tanner, 1986) are given below.

Testes Development

The orchidometer (Prader, 1966) consists of 12 models of rotation ellipsoids with volumes of 1, 2, 3, 4, 5, 6, 8, 10, 12, 15, 20 and 25 ml. The testicular volume recorded was the volume of the ellipsoid that was nearest in volume to that of the testis examined.

Genital Development

Stage 1 (G1). Pre-adolescent. Testes, scrotum and penis are about the same size and in the same proportion as in early childhood.

Stage 2 (G2). Enlargement of scrotum and testes. The skin of the scrotum reddens and changes in texture. Little or no enlargement of penis at this stage.

Stage 3 (G3). Enlargement of penis, which occurs at first mainly in length. Further growth of testes and scrotum.

Stage 4 (G4). Increased size of penis, with growth in breadth and development of glands. Further enlargement of testes and scrotum; increased darkening of scrotal skin.

Stage 5 (G5). Genitalia are adult in size and shape.

Axillary Hair

Stage 1 (Ax1). Pre-adolescent; infantile, no hair.

Stage 2 (Ax2). Sparse hair.

Pubic Hair

Stage 1 (PH1). Pre-adolescent. The vellus over the pubes is not further developed than that over the abdominal wall, i.e., there is no pubic hair.

Stage 2 (PH2). Sparse growth of long, slightly pigmented downy hair, straight or only slightly curled, appearing chiefly at the base of the penis.

Stage 3 (PH3). The hair is considerably darker, coarser and more curled. It spreads sparsely over the junction of the pubes.

Stage 4 (PH4). Hair is now adult type, but the area covered by it is still considerably smaller than in most adults, and it has not spread to the medial surface of the thighs.

Stage 5 (PH5). Hair is adult in quantity and type, distributed in an inverse angle of the classically feminine pattern. Spread to the medial surface of the thighs, but not up linea alba or elsewhere above the base of the inverse triangle.

Skin (Acne)

Stage 1 (S1). Pre-adolescent; no acne.

Stage 2 (S2). Presence of acne.

Voice Change

Stage 1 (V1). Pre-adolescent. The pitch of the voice had not changed noticeably.

Stage 2 (V2). Pubertal voice. The pitch of the voice had changed noticeably but the voice had not yet acquired adult characteristics.

Stage 3 (V3). Adult voice. The pitch of the voice has adult characteristics.

Facial Hair

Stage 1 (FH1). Pre-adolescent; infantile, no hair.

Stage 2 (FH2). Slightly long and pigmented hair at the corners of upper lip.

METHODS OF ANALYSIS

Peak Height Velocity (PHV)

The period of PHV was defined as the 12-month period during which the greatest increase of standing height occurred; the age at PHV was defined as the midpoint of that interval. The estimation of PHV was done by visual inspection of the unsmoothed incremental curves of standing height, which were based on the measurements taken every third month and adjusted to exactly specified target ages, e.g., 10.00 years, 10.25 years and so on (Karlberg *et al.,* 1976; Taranger, 1976).

Statistical Analysis

The age of a subject at the attainment of a specific stage for a given maturity indicator was defined as the midpoint of the interval during which the stage was observed. Those individual ages were used in the calculation of the mean ages and the Pearson's correlation analysis. The age distribution of the attainment of the maturity indicators in relation to the occurrence of peak height velocity was also described as a cumulative percentage. In the calculations of cumulative percentage, the same principles used in the probit analysis (Finney, 1971) were applied.

RESULTS

Age on Reaching Stages

Means and standard deviations of the ages of the attainment of various pubertal events and their association with the age at peak height velocity (PHV) are given in Table 1. The cumulative percentage of boys who have attained a certain maturity indicator in relation to the interval during which PHV occurred is given in Table 2.

There was no boy with signs of pubertal development before the registration at 10 years. There was variation, ranging between five and nine years, in the attainment of the various stages of pubertal development. According to the mean values, testis volume 4, 5, 6, 8, 10 and 12 ml, genital stages 2, 3 and 4, pubic hair stages 2 and 3, pubertal voice V2, axillary hair Ax2 and skin change S2 were attained 2.2 to 0.0 years before the pubertal maximum of growth (PHV), and the remaining indicators were attained 0.1 to 1.8 years after.

On average, the first pubertal sign was testis volume 4 ml at 11.9 years, followed by genital stage 2 at 12.3 years and pubic hair stage 2 and testis volume 5 ml at 12.4 years. At 10 years of age, pubertal signs were observed in a few boys: a testis volume of 4-6 ml, pubic hair stage 2 and genital stage 3. In several boys, the first signs of pubertal development were not observed until 15 years of age.

Table 1. The age at occurrence of stages of the development of secondary sex characteristics in males, and the correlation coefficients between age at attainment of various maturity indicators of secondary sex characteristics and pubertal maximum of growth (PHV). The sequence of occurrence according to mean ages is given.

Stage	Number	Mean	S.D.	Age Range	Sequence	Correlation with PHV
Testis Volume						
4 ml	95	11.9	1.08	9.5-14.5	1	0.80*
5 ml	94	12.4	1.04	9.5-14.5	4	0.85*
6 ml	94	12.7	1.04	9.5-14.5	5	0.87*
8 ml	94	13.1	1.07	10.5-15.5	6	0.85*
10 ml	95	13.5	1.08	10.5-15.5	9	0.84*
12 ml	94	13.9	1.05	11.5-15.5	11	0.79*
15 ml	93	14.4	1.04	11.5-16.5	17	0.72*
20 ml	92	15.3	1.05	11.5-17.5	20	0.55*
25 ml	87	16.3	1.17	13.5-19.5	23	0.47*
Genital Development						
G2	91	12.3	1.16	9.5-14.5	2	0.83*
G3	93	13.1	1.17	9.5-15.5	7	0.91*
G4	96	14.0	1.22	11.5-16.5	12	0.92*
G5	90	15.2	1.36	12.5-19.5	19	0.78*
Axillary Hair						
Ax2	94	14.0	1.43	10.5-19.5	13	0.71*
Pubic Hair						
PH2	96	12.4	1.37	9.5-15.5	3	0.57*
PH3	95	13.4	1.13	10.5-16.5	8	0.86*
PH4	94	14.2	1.20	11.5-16.5	16	0.92*
PH5	90	15.6	1.53	12.5-19.5	21	0.73*
Skin						
S2	86	14.1	1.93	11.5-19.5	15	0.36*
Voice						
V2	98	13.9	0.95	11.5-16.5	10	0.82*
V3	91	15.0	0.91	12.5-17.5	18	0.73*
Facial Hair						
FH2	85	15.9	2.16	12.5-	22	0.52*
Peak Height Velocity (PHV)	105	14.1	1.08	11.5-17.5	14	

*$p < 0.001$

Testis. Testis volume 4 ml was observed between 9.5 and 14.5 years. The earliest boy had a testis volume of 25 ml at 14 years. All except one

Table 2. Cumulative percentage of subjects attaining a certain testes volume (4-25 ml) or a certain stage of a secondary sex characteristic at the end of each annual interval in relation to the interval during which the peak of the pubertal growth spurt occurred.

	Year												
Stage	-5	-4	-3	-2	-1	PHV	+1	+2	+3	+4	+5	+6	+7
Testis Volume													
4 ml	-	3.2	19.6	79.8	97.8	100	-	-	-	-	-	-	-
5 ml	-	2.2	4.1	51.5	94.9	100	-	-	-	-	-	-	-
6 ml	-	-	2.1	38.4	86.9	100	-	-	-	-	-	-	-
8 ml	-	-	-	20.2	62.6	99.0	100	-	-	-	-	-	-
10 ml	-	-	-	6.1	46.5	91.7	100	-	-	-	-	-	-
12 ml	-	-	-	3.0	28.3	76.0	97.8	100	-	-	-	-	-
15 ml	-	-	-	3.0	14.1	52.1	85.6	100	-	-	-	-	-
20 ml	-	-	-	-	6.1	24.0	54.4	82.3	93.5	100	-	-	-
25 ml	-	-	-	-	1.0	5.2	25.6	60.0	84.4	90.2	100	-	-
Genital Development													
G2	-	1.0	17.7	55.6	92.9	100	-	-	-	-	-	-	-
G3	-	-	-	13.1	70.4	100	-	-	-	-	-	-	-
G4	-	-	-	-	15.3	82.4	99.0	100	-	-	-	-	-
G5	-	-	-	-	2.0	18.8	65.7	94.6	98.9	100	-	-	-
Axillary Hair													
Ax2	-	-	1.0	6.9	25.7	68.0	90.8	98.0	100	-	-	-	-
Pubic Hair													
PH2	2.0	10.7	23.2	40.0	78.2	100	-	-	-	-	-	-	-
PH3	-	-	-	11.0	41.4	96.9	100	-	-	-	-	-	-
PH4	-	-	-	-	12.2	71.1	100	-	-	-	-	-	-
PH5	-	-	-	-	-	16.7	50.5	80.4	95.6	100	-	-	-
Skin													
S2	-	-	1.0	11.9	29.6	61.6	76.3	84.2	90.5	97.8	-	-	-
Voice													
V2	-	-	-	2.9	23.5	86.1	100	-	-	-	-	-	-
V3	-	-	-	1.0	2.0	25.0	76.8	99.0	100	-	-	-	-
Facial Hair													
FH2	-	-	-	-	3.0	17.0	41.0	64.8	76.1	88.4	93.0	95.3	100

boy had a testis volume of 25 ml at 18 years; that boy had a testis volume of 25 ml at 21 years. The increase in volume from 4 to 25 ml occurred, on the average, in 4.7 years, between 11.6 and 16.3 years.

Genitalia. The change from G2 to G5 occurred in nearly 3 years, from 12.3 to 15.2 years. The change in genital development started between 9.5 and 14.5 years and was completed between 12.5 and 19.5 years.

Axillary Hair. Sparse axillary hair (Ax2) was observed for the first time between 10.5 and 19.5 years.

Pubic Hair. The change from PH2 to PH5 occurred in 3.2 years, from 12.4 to 15.6 years. Pubic hair became visible between 9.5 to 15.5 years, and had reached its adult characteristics between 12.5 and 19.5 years.

Skin. Acne was registered in 98% of the boys followed, and was observed for the first time between 11.5 and 19.5 years.

Voice Change. The change from pubertal voice to adult voice took about one year, from 14 to 15 years. The pubertal voice (V2) was attained between 11.5 and 16.5 years, and adult voice (V3) between 12.5 and 17.5 years.

Facial Hair. The first sign of facial hair was observed between 12.5 and 19.5 years for the majority of boys and for 6% (5 of 90 boys) between 21 and 25 years.

Peak Height Velocity. Peak height velocity occurred between 11.5 and 17.5 years.

Interrelationships Between Ages of Attainment of Maturity Indicators of Secondary Sex Characteristics and PHV

Testis and PHV. According to the mean values, testis volumes 4-12 ml were attained before and testis volumes 15-25 ml after PHV. The correlation coefficients between the testis volumes and PHV were moderate or high (between 0.47 and 0.87; Table 1), with the lower correlations being observed for the larger testis volumes.

A testis volume of at least 8 ml was achieved before or at PHV by all boys except one (Table 2). Testis volumes 10 and 12 ml were attained in about 95% of the boys from 1 year before to 1 year after PHV. A testis volume of 20 or 25 ml was only attained before PHV by 5% and 1% of the boys, respectively.

Genital Development and PHV. According to the mean values, stages G2 and G3 were attained before, and G4 and G5 after, PHV. The correlation coefficients between the genital stages and PHV were high, being 0.78 to 0.92 (Table 1).

G3 was attained before or at PHV (Table 2). G4 was attained from one year before to one year after PHV, and the final stage (G5) was attained at or after PHV in 98% of the subjects.

Axillary hair and PHV are, on average, attained at the same age. The correlation coefficients between PHV and this initial stage of axillary hair (Ax2) was 0.71 (Table 1). The initial sign of axillary hair was observed from 3 years before to 3 years after PHV (Table 2).

Pubic Hair and PHV. According to the mean values, PH2 and PH3 were attained before, and PH4 and PH5 after, PHV. The correlation coefficients between the initial and final stages and PHV were moderate, but for the intermediate stages and PHV they were high (Table 1).

PH2 was attained before or at PHV (Table 2) as was PH3 in 97% of the boys. In all subjects, PH4 was attained from 1 year before to 1 year after PHV. PH5 was attained at or after PHV.

Skin Change and PHV. Skin change (S2) occurred, according to the mean value, at the same age as PHV, but the association between the two parameters was low (Table 1). The initial sign of skin change was observed from 4 years before to 4 years after PHV (Table 2).

Voice Change and PHV. On the average, pubertal voice (V2) was attained just before PHV and adult voice (V3) a year after it, and the association between the stages of voice change and PHV was high (Table 1). In 97% of the subjects, pubertal voice V2 was acquired from 1 year before to 1 year after PHV. V3 was acquired at or within 2 years after PHV in 97% of the subjects.

Facial Hair and PHV. The first sign of facial hair (FH2) was observed almost 2 years after PHV (Table 1). Only 3% had reached FH2 before PHV, and some reached it 7 years after PHV (Table 2).

DISCUSSION

To study the relationships between developmental and growth events such as those examined in this study, it is necessary to collect data by means of longitudinal studies of a sufficiently large number of subjects followed from an age preceding any sign of puberty to an age when all have reached the final stages of pubertal development. In samples that have not been followed for a sufficiently long period, early and/or late maturers are apt to be under-represented. Furthermore, in any longitudinal study a substantial number of dropouts is inevitable. Since this number increases with time, the proportion of early, average and late maturers is very likely to be biased. As a rule, this bias is not taken into account in the statistical analysis. Consequently, the representativeness of the results of the previous studies is often uncertain. The present sample is representative for a Swedish urban community; the dropouts are few and their growth pattern did not differ from that of the total sample (Karlberg *et al.,* 1976). Owing to the few dropouts and the small number of missing examinations, the pubertal maximum of growth and the maturity indicators of secondary sex characteristics were determined in a very large proportion of the original sample. As shown by the ranges given for the investigated parameters (Table 1), both early and late maturers were included. As six of the 23 pubertal events were not attained in all subjects by the annual examinations up to 18 years, there might be a small overestimation of the mean ages for some of the late occurring indicators. Ideally, a study of development of the secondary sex characteristics should cover the age period from 9 to about 23 years by annual examinations.

The Timing of Secondary Sex Characteristics

In the present study, peak height velocity (PHV) occurred, on the average, at 14 years, which is in agreement with other contemporary studies (for review, see Marshall and Tanner, 1986).

Testicular Volume. In general, the testicular volumes found in the present study were in agreement with those reported from a large cross-sectional Dutch study (van Wieringen *et al.,* 1971). The strikingly low values in a longitudinal study of Swiss boys (Largo and Prader, 1983) may be explained by differing use of the orchidometer and approach to reading measurements compared to other studies. In the present study the nearest volume was recorded, while in the Swiss study the volume recorded was equal to or less than the true volume. The orchidometer in the Dutch study was calibrated to smaller intervals, especially in the upper range. In the present study a testicular volume of at least 25 ml was recorded at 21 years in all subjects. At about 20 years of age an average testicular volume of 24 ml was reported from the Dutch study (van Wieringen *et al.,* 1971) and 19 ml from the Swiss study (Largo and Prader, 1983).

Genital Development and Pubic Hair. The attainment of most of the investigated stages were in general agreement with other contemporary European studies (Marshall and Tanner, 1970; van Wieringen *et al.,* 1971; Largo and Prader, 1983).

Skin, Voice Change, Axillary Hair, Facial Hair. Comparison with other European studies is difficult due to the paucity of reports.

Secondary Sex Characteristics and Pubertal Maximum of Growth. A high association was found between the attainment of several stages of secondary sex characteristics and pubertal maximum of growth (Table 1). A direct comparison with other European studies can only be done to a limited extent, because some of those studies do not include all of the parameters examined here, or the results presented are incomplete (e.g., Marshall and Tanner, 1970; Largo and Prader, 1983).

Genital development seems more advanced at pubertal maximum in the Swedish (Table 2) and English boys (Marshall and Tanner, 1970) than in the Swiss boys (Largo and Prader, 1983), although this may be attributable to variations in the devices used and methods of reading measurements between the Swiss study and the others. A similar pattern was observed between pubic hair and pubertal maximum. This is the first study to describe the relationship in time between specific secondary sex characteristics such as axillary hair, facial hair, skin and peak height velocity (Tables 1, 2).

Clinical Implications

It has been shown that the skeletal contribution to the change from a Class II to a Class I dental arch relationship, especially in male patients, is most pronounced at PHV or during the year following (Hägg *et al.*, 1987; Hägg and Pancherz, 1988). Estimation of PHV in the individual patient, therefore, seems likely to be of value, especially when the patient has a severe maxillomandibular skeletal discrepancy. The best method for estimating PHV is to analyze the individual's velocity or distance curves of standing height (Björk, 1972; Pancherz and Hägg, 1985; Hägg *et al.*, 1987; Karlberg, 1987; Malmgren *et al.*, 1987; Hägg and Pancherz, 1988). Since longitudinal data of standing height is seldom available in the clinical context, one has to rely on indirect methods, such as the use of hand-wrist radiographs (e.g., Helm *et al.*, 1971; Hägg and Taranger, 1982; Hägg *et al.*, 1987; Hägg and Pancherz, 1988) and/or evaluation of secondary sex characteristics. The present study shows that indicators such as, for example, testicular volumes of 12 to 15 ml, genital stage 4, pubic hair stage 4 and pubertal voice stage 2 do indicate that a male is in a very intensive period of growth. Such information, which could be obtained through cooperation with a patient's physician, can be used in orthodontic treatment planning for male patients with severe skeletal problems.

CONCLUSIONS

1. There is great individual variation in the timing of peak height velocity and the stage of secondary sex characteristics in males.

2. There is a high association in the occurrence of certain stages of development in the secondary sex characteristics and the pubertal maximum of growth in males.

3. Certain stages of development in the secondary sex characteristics seem to be accurate indirect tools to estimate the most intensive period of facial growth in males.

ACKNOWLEDGMENTS

The present study was supported by grants from the Faculty of Medicine, University of Göteborg; the Faculty of Odontology, Malmö, University of Lund; the Swedish Medical Research Council, Stockholm; and the Swedish Dental Society, Stockholm, Sweden.

REFERENCES

Björk, A. Timing of orthodontic interceptive measures based on stages of maturation. Trans. Eur. Orthod. Soc. *48:*61-74, 1972.

Björk, A. and S. Helm. Prediction of the age of maximum pubertal growth in body height. Angle Orthod. *37:*134-143, 1967.

Finney, D.J. *Probit Analysis.* 3rd. Ed., Cambridge University Press, Cambridge, 1971.

George, D.I. Elevations of the pituitary gonadotropins associated with the onset of puberty. In: *Craniofacial Growth During Adolescence.* D.S. Carlson and K.A. Ribbens (Eds.), Monograph 20, Craniofacial Growth Series, Center for Human Growth and Development, The University of Michigan, Ann Arbor, 1987.

Hägg, U. The pubertal growth spurt and maturity indicators of dental, skeletal and pubertal development. A prospective longitudinal study of Swedish urban children. Doctoral dissertation, University of Lund, Malmö, Sweden, 1980.

Hägg, U., H. Pancherz and J. Taranger. Pubertal growth and orthodontic treatment. In: *Craniofacial Growth During Adolescence.* D.S. Carlson and K.A. Ribbens (Eds.), Monograph 20, Craniofacial Growth Series, Center for Human Growth and Development, The University of Michigan, Ann Arbor, 1987.

Hägg, U. and H. Pancherz. Dentofacial orthopaedics in relation to chronological age, growth period and skeletal development. An analysis of 72 male patients with Class II, division 1 malocclusion treated with the Herbst appliance. Eur. J. Orthod. *10:*169-176, 1988.

Hägg, U. and J. Taranger. Maturation indicators and the pubertal growth spurt. Am. J. Orthod. *82:*299-309, 1982.

Karlberg, J. Modelling of human growth. Doctoral dissertation, University of Göteborg, Sweden, 1987.

Karlberg, P., J. Taranger, I. Engström, J. Karlberg, T. Landstrom, H. Lichtenstein and I. Svennberg-Redegren. Physical growth from birth to 16 years and the longitudinal outcome of the study during the same age period. Acta Paediatr. Scand. Suppl. *258:*7-76, 1976.

Largo, R.H. and A. Prader. Pubertal development in Swiss boys. Helvet. Paediatr. Acta *38:*211-228, 1983.

Malmgren, O., J. ömblus, U. Hägg and H. Pancherz. Treatment with an orthopedic appliance system in relation to treatment intensity and growth periods. Am. J. Orthod. *91:*143-151, 1987.

Marshall, W.A. and J.M. Tanner. Variations in pattern of pubertal changes in boys. Arch. Dis. Child. *45:*13-23, 1970.

Marshall, W.A. and J.M. Tanner. Puberty. In: *Human Growth 2.* F. Falkner and J.M. Tanner (Eds.), Ballière Tindall, London, 1986.

Pancherz, H. and U. Hägg. Dentofacial orthopedics in relation to somatic maturation. Am. J. Orthod. *88:*273-287, 1985.

Pancherz, H., O. Malmgren, U. Hägg, J. ömblus and K. Hansen. Class II correction in Herbst and Bass therapy. A comparative study considering somatic maturity and skeletofacial morphology. Eur. J. Orthod. Accepted for publication, 1988.

Prader, A. Testicular size: Assessment and clinical importance. Triangle *7:*240, 1966.

Tanner, J.M. *Growth at Adolescence.* 2nd Ed., Blackwell Scientific Publications, Oxford, 1962.

Taranger, J. Evaluation of biological maturation by means of maturity criteria. Acta Paediatr. Scand. Suppl. *258:*77-82, 1976.

van Wieringen, J.C., F. Wafelbakker, H.P. Verbrugge and J.H. de Hass. *Growth Diagrams 1965–Netherlands.* Wolters-Noordhoff Publishing, Groningen, 1971.

Weiner, J.S. and J.A. Lourie. *Human Biology: A Guide to Field Methods.* Blackwell, Oxford, 1969.

RESPONSIVENESS OF ALVEOLAR BONE TO ORTHODONTIC TREATMENT IN ADULT PATIENTS

Jeanne J. Stutzmann
Alexandre G. Petrovic

The response of alveolar bone to physiologically- and orthodontically-induced tooth movement has already been studied both in humans and in animals. These studies have been based mostly on histologic, cytochemical and immunocytochemical descriptions; only a few have dealt with quantification of alveolar bone formation and/or resorption.[1]

The frequency of orthodontic treatment in adults has increased considerably during the last decade, primarily for three reasons. First, many adults are now seeking treatment for maxillomandibular discrepancies and dental malocclusions that originated in childhood and should have been corrected at that time. Second, there are conditions that originate in the adult, for example, crowding as the result of a new neuromuscular balance, that require treatment. Third, orthodontic treatment is increasingly necessary in adults in order to make preprosthetic corrections.

In our previous investigations (Stutzmann and Petrovic, 1984), we provided quantitative estimates of the spontaneous and the therapeutically-induced variations in the turnover rate of alveolar bone collected in 11 to 13-year-old patients. It was determined in that study that the alveolar bone turnover rate varied as a function of (1) the localization of the alveolar bone (mesial vs. distal), (2) the type of mandibular rotation (anterior vs. posterior), (3) the circadian timing of the extraction, and (4) the season (spring vs. autumn). In that study, we also demonstrated that

1. Stein and Weinmann, 1925; Reitan, 1947, 1951, 1960, 1964, 1974; Macapanpan *et al.*, 1954; Storey, 1955; Graber *et al.*, 1967; Baumrind, 1969; Giannelly, 1969; Baumrind and Buck, 1970; Kvam, 1970, 1972; Klingler, 1971; Baron, 1973; Markostamos and Baron, 1973; Markostamos, 1974; Rygh, 1972, 1973, 1974, 1984, 1986; Rygh and Selvig, 1973; Kurihara, 1977; Fruge *et al.*, 1980; Davidovitch *et al.*, 1980, 1984; Roberts and Chase, 1981; Lilja *et al.*, 1983; Yamasaki *et al.*, 1984; Rygh *et al.*, 1986; Melsen, 1986; Shanfeld *et al.*, 1986; Stark and Sinclair, 1987; Caton *et al.*, 1987.

light forces applied for only part of the day are the most efficient means of increasing the alveolar bone turnover rate.

The purpose of this paper is to address three questions regarding tooth movement and alveolar bone turnover rate in adult patients:

1. What is the level of the alveolar bone turnover rate in 20 to 25-year-old male patients compared to that of three other age groups (8 to 9; 11 to 13; 16 to 17)?
2. Do the physiologic variations detected in 11 to 13-year-old boys persist when the individual becomes an adult (i.e., reaches the end of growth, not sexual maturity)?
3. To what extent is it possible to therapeutically modify the alveolar bone turn-over rate in the young adult, by means of various orthodontic forces?

METHODS

The quantitative estimation method involving the use of organ culture for analysis of the human alveolar bone turnover rate and the general procedure used in the current study were described in detail previously (Stutzmann and Petrovic, 1984, 1986).

First Experimental Series (Table 1)

Alveolar bone specimens were collected from 120 male subjects with Class II malocclusions, between the ages of 7 and 25 years, during extraction of mandibular first premolars as part of orthodontic treatment. The subjects were divided into four groups of 30 according to age: 7 to 8 years of age, 11 to 13 years of age, 16 to 17 years of age, and 20 to 25 years of age. All the alveolar bone specimens were placed in organ culture for 72 hours. Bone formation rate was estimated by measuring the alkaline phenylphosphatase activity. Bone mineralization rate was determined by measuring the uptake of ^{45}Ca. Bone resorption rate was determined by measuring β–glucuronidase and acid phenylphosphatase activities.

Second Experimental Series

Alveolar bone fragments were collected from 95 male subjects, aged 20 to 25 years, between April 1 and July 1 (Group I) and from 70 male subjects in the same age group between October 15 and January 15

Table 1. Research design.

	Pretreatment Cases	Cases after Onset of Treatment		
April 1-July 1 Extractions (N = 95)		Light Intermittent	Heavy Intermittent	Light Continuous
Posterior "inclination" of mandible (IP)	35	35	-	-
Anterior "inclination" of mandible (IA)	60	35	10	15
October 15-January 15 Extractions (N = 70)				
Posterior "inclination" of mandible (IIP)	35	-	-	-
Anterior "inclination" of mandible (IIA)	35	-	-	-

(Group II). The patients all had Class II malocclusions. Various subgroups were constituted according to the research design (Table 1).

The first mandibular premolar was extracted and the contiguous mesially- and distally-located alveolar bone was collected on one side (either left or right) before orthodontic treatment was begun. The specimens were immediately organ-cultured for 72 hours and measured for the parameters mentioned above.

After the premolar extraction, only the subjects from Group I (spring group) were fitted with Class II elastics on the contralateral side of the mandible (either right or left). Mesially-directed forces were applied for 21 days as follows: 35 individuals in Group IA (individuals with "anteriorly inclined"[2] mandibles) and 35 individuals in Group IP (individuals with "posteriorly inclined" mandibles) were treated with a light (75 to 50 g), intermittent (14 hours daily) force; 10 individuals in Group IA were treated with a heavy (275 to 175 g), intermittent (14 hours daily) force; and 15 individuals in Group IA were treated with a light (75 to 50 g), continuous force.

2. Strictly, growth rotation of the mandible refers to the time-related variations occurring during the growth of the individual. When dealing with basic features of the individual, the word "inclination" is perhaps more appropriate.

Table 2. Variations of the human alveolar bone turnover rate as a function of the age of the patient.

^{45}Ca uptake (c.p.m.)

Age (years)	N	Median	Range	Multiple comparisons[1] II	III	IV
I. 7-8	30	10,982	7,636-15,260	NS[2]	***	***
II. 11-13	30	10,549	4,738-19,327		***	***
III. 16-17	30	2,523	1,025-8,184			NS
IV. 20-25	30	2,705	1,319-8,043			

T = 82.74 with 3 degrees of freedom.
Approximation by χ^2 distribution: $p < 0.0001$.

Acid phenylphosphatase activity (e.u.)

Age (years)	N	Median	Range	Multiple comparisons[1] II	III	IV
I. 7-8	30	11.55	7.82 -15.38	*	***	***
II. 11-13	30	13.22	6.42- 21.36		***	***
III. 16-17	30	3.78	1.80-10.81			*
IV. 20-25	30	5.60	2.67-13.29			

T = 76.166 with 3 degrees of freedom.
Approximation by χ^2 distribution: $p < 0.0001$.

[1]Kruskal-Wallis test: p is the probability that the statement "The levels of alveolar bone turn-over will vary for different age groups" is wrong.
[2]NS: not significant; * difference significant at 0.05; ** difference significant at 0.01; *** difference significant at 0.001

After the 21-day orthodontic treatment, the remaining first mandibular premolar, i.e., on the opposite side, was extracted and contiguous mesially- and distally-located alveolar bone fragments were collected, cultured as previously described, and analyzed. The adult patients were then treated with the Edgewise appliance. Clinical effectiveness was evaluated semi-quantitatively by the orthodontist for each individual patient after one year of treatment using a scale of 0 (barely effective) to +++ (highly effective). A double-blind study design was used.

These procedures provided the following information for individual patients:

1. The basic biologic alveolar bone turnover rate.

2. The alveolar bone turnover rate after a 21-day treatment with Class II elastics.

3. The clinical effectiveness estimated by the orthodontist after one year of Edgewise treatment.

RESULTS AND DISCUSSION

The statistical analysis of the data collected following organ culture shows that the various experimental populations were not distributed normally. Hence, it was necessary to use nonparametric statistical tests in this analysis (Siegel, 1956; Conover, 1980). In order to compare two independent samples, the Mann-Witney U-test was employed; for multiple comparisons, the Kruskal-Wallis test was used. The Wilcoxon matched-pairs signed-rank test was used to compare two related samples.

Spontaneous Turnover Rate of the Alveolar Bone

For a given individual, the level of the alveolar bone turnover rate is defined, operationally, as the mean of the values of the mesial and the distal sides. The alveolar bone turnover rate presented a number of variations.

Variations as a Function of the Age of the Patients (Table 2). The ^{45}Ca and the acid phenylphosphatase activity were much higher in the 7 to 8-year-old boys and in the 11 to 13-year-old boys than in the 16 to 17-year-old boys and in the 20 to 25-year-old patients. Nevertheless, it must be pointed out that:

1. The ^{45}Ca uptake in alveolar bone collected in 7 to 8-year-old boys was not significantly different from that of alveolar bone collected in 11 to 13-year-old boys.

2. The ^{45}Ca uptake in alveolar bone collected in 20 to 25-year-old male patients was not significantly different from that of alveolar bone collected in 16 to 17-year-old male patients.

3. The acid phenylphosphatase activity was significantly higher in alveolar bone collected in 11 to 13-year-old boys than in alveolar bone collected in 7 to 8-year-old patients.

Table 3. Variations of the human alveolar bone turnover rate as a function of the alveolar bone location (mesial vs. distal) referring to the extracted premolar.

Alkaline phenylphosphatase activity (e.u.)		N	Median	Range	Value of z[1]
Anterior	Distal	70	37.7	13.4-107.4	-2.9
	Mesial	70	38.9	16.2-123.2	p = 0.004 M > D
Posterior	Distal	70	25.9	6.3-92.8	-4.49
	Mesial	70	29.1	7.2-99.3	p < 0.0001 M > D
^{45}Ca uptake (c.p.m.)					
Anterior	Distal	70	3,470	1,307-8,678	0.63
	Mesial	70	3,553	1,373-9,137	p = 0.2643 NS
Posterior	Distal	70	2,080	1,052-8,251	-4.08
	Mesial	70	1,927	1,158-7,929	p < 0.0001 D > M
β-glucuronidase activity (F.u.)					
Anterior	Distal	70	10.03	5.48-27.02	-1.47
	Mesial	70	10.18	5.21-26.31	p = 0.0708 NS
Posterior	Distal	70	8.49	5.07-27.84	-0.56
	Mesial	70	8.41	5.45-29.15	p = 0.2877 NS
Acid phenylphosphatase activity (e.u.)					
Anterior	Distal	70	5.28	2.33-13.94	-2.45
	Mesial	70	5.96	2.31-13.68	p = 0.0071 D > M
Posterior	Distal	70	5.04	2.14-13.85	-3.91
	Mesial	70	4.77	2.31-13.25	p < 0.0001 D > M

[1]Wilcoxon matched-pairs signed-ranks test

Anterior = mandible in anterior inclination.

Posterior = mandible in posterior inclination.

4. The acid phenylphosphatase activity was also significantly higher in alveolar bone collected in 20 to 25-year-old patients than in alveolar bone collected in 16 to 17-year-old patients.

The higher value of acid phenylphosphatase activity was not significantly matched by a corresponding increase in ^{45}Ca in either set of comparisons (i.e., 7-8 vs. 11-13 and 16-17 vs. 20-25 year age groups). So far we have no valid explanation for this finding. Further investigations are necessary.

In our sample, a significant decrease in alveolar bone turnover rate occurred between age 13 and 16.

Variations as a Function of the Alveolar Bone Location (distal vs. mesial) Referring to the Extracted Premolar. The results of the Wilcoxon matched-pairs signed-rank test lead to the following findings (Table 3). First, regardless of the inclination of the mandible, the alkaline phenylphosphatase activity was higher on the mesial side than on the distal side. Second, the acid phenylphosphatase activity was higher on the distal side than on the mesial side, and no statistically significant difference was detected between the mesial and distal sides for β-glucuronidase activity. As for ^{45}Ca uptake, the result varied as a function of the inclinational type; in the anteriorly inclined mandible no statistically significant difference was detected between the mesial and the distal side, whereas in the posteriorly inclined mandible, the ^{45}Ca uptake was slightly higher on the distal than on the mesial side. In general, according to the alveolar bone turnover rate on the distal and on the mesial side, the first mandibular premolar did not undergo a significant sagittal movement. Indeed, the observed small differences, even when statistically significant, were actually in the range of individual variation. It should be recalled that the situation is different in the growing child, when the distalization of the first premolar is primarily associated with an anteriorly rotating mandible whereas the mesialization of the first premolar is generally associated with the posteriorly rotating mandible (Stutzmann and Petrovic, 1984).

Variations as a Function of the Mandibular Inclination (anterior vs. posterior). The Mann-Witney U-test (Table 4) indicated that the alkaline phenylphosphatase activity, the ^{45}Ca uptake, and the acid phenylphosphatase activity were significantly higher in the alveolar bone originating from anteriorly inclined mandibles than from posteriorly inclined mandibles. The difference for β-glucuronidase activity was not statistically significant, although there was a clear tendency for it to be higher

Table 4. Variations of human alveolar bone turnover rate as a function of the inclination of the mandible (anterior vs. posterior).

Alkaline phenylphosphatase activity (e.u.)

	N	Median	Range	Value of z[1]
Anterior	70	37.8	16.0-115.3	2.57
Posterior	70	27.3	7.1-96.2	$p = 0.005$ **

Uptake of ^{45}Ca (c.p.m.)

	N	Median	Range	Value of z[1]
Anterior	70	3,455	1,340-8,907	4.01
Posterior	70	1,991	1,174-8,053	$p < 0.001$ ***

β-glucuronidase activity (F.u.)

	N	Median	Range	Value of z[1]
Anterior	70	10.09	5.34-26.66	1.33
Posterior	70	8.68	5.26-28.49	$p = 0.092$ NS

Acid phenylphosphatase activity (e.u.)

	N	Median	Range	Value of z[1]
Anterior	70	6.20	2.46-13.76	2.07
Posterior	70	4.95	2.22-13.52	$p = 0.019$ *

[1]Mann-Whitney U test

Anterior = mandible in anterior inclination

Posterior = mandible in posterior inclination

[2]NS: not significant; * difference significant at 0.05; ** difference significant at 0.01; *** difference significant at 0.001

in the anteriorly inclined mandible. In other words, in this respect, there was no difference between the data obtained in the young adults and the data obtained in the child.

Variations as a Function of the Season (spring vs. autumn). The statistical analysis of the results (Table 5) shows that β-glucuronidase activ-

Table 5. Variations of human alveolar bone turnover rate as a function of the season (spring vs. autumn).

Alkaline phenylphosphatase activity (e.u.)

	N	Median	Range	Value of z[1]
Spring	70	35.6	12.6-115.3	1.85
Autumn	70	30.2	7.1-77.6	p = 0.063
				NS

Uptake of ^{45}Ca (c.p.m.)

	N	Median	Range	Value of z[1]
Spring	70	3,239	1,445-8,907	1.65
Autumn	70	2,574	1,174-8,053	p = 0.0976
				NS

β-glucuronidase activity (F.u.)

	N	Median	Range	Value of z[1]
Spring	70	11.22	6.03-28.49	2.0692
Autumn	70	8.68	5.26-24.72	p = 0.0385
				*

Acid phenylphosphatase activity (e.u.)

	N	Median	Range	Value of z[1]
Spring	70	6.59	2.51-13.76	2.9048
Autumn	70	5.05	2.22-13.52	p = 0.004
				**

[1]Mann-Whitney U test
Spring = alveolar bone collected between April 1 and July 1
Autumn = alveolar bone collected between October 15 and January 15
[2]NS: not significant; * difference significant at 0.05; ** difference significant at 0.01; *** difference significant at 0.001

ity and acid phenylphosphatase activity were significantly higher in the alveolar bone specimens collected between April 1 and July 1 than in the alveolar bone specimens collected between October 15 and January 15. The alkaline phenylphosphatase activity and the uptake of ^{45}Ca appeared to be higher in spring than in autumn, but no statistically significant difference was detected. Once again, therefore, the results obtained in the young adults are basically similar to the results obtained in the growing child.

Therapeutically-Induced Variations of the Human Alveolar Bone Turnover Rate

The effects of a Class II elastic treatment on the alveolar bone turnover rate can be represented for each individual patient, by calculation of the difference between the value estimated on one side before the onset of the treatment and the value estimated on the opposite side after a 21-day treatment. The median of the calculated differences corresponds to the effect of the treatment for the three research groups (light intermittent forces, heavy intermittent forces, and light continuous forces; Table 6).

Whatever the intensity and the daily duration of the applied mesially-directed orthodontic force, the alveolar bone resorption was always increased in a highly significant way on the mesial side and the alveolar bone formation was increased on the distal side. However, the magnitude of these increases varied with the intensity (light vs. heavy forces) and with the daily duration (intermittent vs. continuous forces) of the application. Indeed, the observed increase of both the bone resorption rate on the mesial side and the bone formation rate on the distal side was highest with light and intermittent forces, and lowest with light and continuous forces (Table 6); thus, when a 50 to 75 g force was applied, the intermittent treatment always appeared to be more effective than the continuous treatment; statistically, however, the light and intermittent forces presented only a tendency to be more effective than the light and continuous forces. This is probably due to the small sample size.

In addition, regardless of the season, the orthodontically-induced increase of the bone formation rate was statistically (but not necessarily in each individual case) higher in the anteriorly inclined mandible than in the posteriorly inclined mandible (Table 7). As for the parameters of bone resorption, a difference was only detected in spring: this difference was significant for β-glucuronidase activity and was only indicative for acid phenylphosphatase activity. As previously mentioned, light and intermittent forces have a less deleterious effect on periodontal tissue and on local circulation than do heavy and continuously applied forces (Stutzmann *et al.,* 1979; Stutzmann and Petrovic, 1984). As a matter of course, local cell multiplication and cell differentiation are less affected by light and intermittent forces. But previous research findings (Lemoine and Petrovic, 1969; Lemoine *et al.,* 1970; Stutzmann *et al.,* 1979, 1980) brought to light another factor: the increased alveolar bone resorption rate and the increased alveolar bone formation rate, as produced orthodontically, involve cells of extrinsic origin (circulating monocyte-type cells). Kurihara (1977) and Rygh and colleagues' (1986) findings seem to corroborate our observations, at least to some extent.

This extrinsic contribution of bone-resorptive and bone-forming cell precursors may account, in part, for the effectiveness of light over heavy and intermittent over continuous orthodontic forces in tooth movement. Indeed, because they have a less damaging effect on circulation, light and intermittent forces allow for a greater local blood supply in mononuclear bone resorptive and bone forming cell precursors of extrinsic origin.

When biological findings and clinical evaluation of the treatment effectiveness were compared (Table 8), a parallel was detected between the level of biological alveolar bone turnover rate, the level of the alveolar bone responsiveness rate to the 21-day Class II elastic treatment and the clinical effectiveness as assessed by the orthodontist one year after the start of treatment. The higher the biological alveolar bone turnover rate was, the higher the alveolar bone responsiveness rate and the higher the clinical effectiveness.

The analysis of Table 8 shows that clinical effectiveness is greater in patients with anteriorly inclining mandibles (where the physiologic alveolar bone turnover rate and the responsiveness rate were higher) than in patients with posteriorly inclining mandibles. Indeed, in the group with anteriorly inclining mandibles, the treatment was barely efficient in only 10 patients, whereas in the group with posteriorly inclining mandibles, 24 patients had a barely efficient treatment.

CONCLUDING REMARKS

The quantitative estimation of the alveolar bone turnover rate allows for several specific conclusions.

1. In young adult male patients, the parameters of bone formation and bone resorption were higher in the anteriorly inclining mandible than in the posteriorly inclining mandible and were higher in spring than in autumn.

Table 6. Variations of the human alveolar bone turnover rate during treatment with Class II elastics (21 day) as a function of the intensity and daily duration of the applied force.

Distal Side: Alveolar Bone Formation

Alkaline phenylphosphatase activity (e.u.)

Force (mesially-directed)	*N*	Median of differences between "After minus Before" treatment	Range of differences between "After minus Before" treatment	Multiple comparisons[1] *H.I.*	*L.C.*
Light intermittent (L.I.)	35	46.1	9.1-255.8	NS	*
Heavy intermittent (H.I.)	10	42.5	22.0-93.8		NS
Light continuous (L.C.)	15	29.7	12.9-114.9		

T = 5.73404 with 2 degrees of freedom
Approximation by χ^2 distribution: p = 0.0569

^{45}Ca uptake (c.p.m.)

Force (mesially-directed)	*N*	Median of differences between "After minus Before" treatment	Range of differences between "After minus Before" treatment	Multiple comparisons[1] *H.I.*	*L.C.*
Light intermittent (L.I.)	35	3,519	1,489-10,715	*	***
Heavy intermittent (H.I.)	10	3,161	1,050-3,907		NS
Light continuous (L.C.)	15	2,330	655-4,754		

T = 13.72417 with 2 degrees of freedom
Approximation by χ^2 distribution: p = 0.0010

Table 6. Continued.

Mesial Side: Alveolar Bone Resorption

β-glucuronidase activity (F.u.)

Force (mesially-directed)	*N*	Median of differences between "After minus Before" treatment	Range of differences between "After minus Before" treatment	Multiple comparisons[1] *H.I.*	Multiple comparisons[1] *L.C.*
Light intermittent (L.I.)	35	25.98	5.74-49.35	*	***
Heavy intermittent (H.I.)	10	10.31	2.72-17.74		NS
Light continuous (L.C.)	15	8.95	3.20-15.31		

T = 21.50753 with 2 degrees of freedom
Approximation by χ^2 distribution: $p < 0.0001$

Acid phenylphosphatase activity (e.u.)

Force (mesially-directed)	*N*	Median of differences between "After minus Before" treatment	Range of differences between "After minus Before" treatment	Multiple comparisons[1] *H.I.*	Multiple comparisons[1] *L.C.*
Light intermittent (L.I.)	35	11.65	2.21-23.29	**	***
Heavy intermittent (H.I.)	10	3.66	1.34-17.17		NS
Light continuous (L.C.)	15	2.70	0.43-7.10		

T = 21.40458 with 2 degrees of freedom
Approximation by χ^2 distribution: $p < 0.0001$

[1]Kruskal-Wallis test: p is the probability that the statement "The effects of a 21-day Class II elastic treatment on bone formation and bone resorption will vary according to the intensity and daily duration of the treatment" is wrong.

Table 7. Effects of a 21-day Class II elastic treatment (light intermittent force) as a function of the mandible inclination and of the season.

Distal Side: Alveolar Bone Formation

Alkaline phenylphosphatase activity (e.u.)

Season	Inclination	*N*	Median	Range	Multiple comparisons[1] II	III	IV
I. Spring	Anterior	35	46.1	9.1–255.8	***	NS	***
II.	Posterior	35	27.6	5.0–156.6		**	NS
III. Autumn	Anterior	35	41.7	21.4–166.6			***
IV.	Posterior	35	14.4	2.2–152.8			

T = 29.649 with 3 degrees of freedom
Approximation by χ^2 distribution: $p < 0.0001$

^{45}Ca uptake (c.p.m.)

Season	Inclination	*N*	Median	Range	Multiple comparisons[1] II	III	IV
I. Spring	Anterior	35	3,519	1,489–10,715	***	***	***
II.	Posterior	35	685	-105–9,696		***	*
III. Autumn	Anterior	35	2,086	-139–10,302			***
IV.	Posterior	35	417	-98–7,053			

T = 61.016 with 3 degrees of freedom
Approximation by χ^2 distribution: $p < 0.0001$

Basically, these results were similar to those obtained in the 11 to 13-year-old boys. However, the turnover rate of the alveolar bone decreased sharply between the ages of 13 to 16.

2. In young adult male patients, no systematic difference was detected between the alveolar bone turnover rate on the distal and the mesial sides. This finding is not unexpected because the growth of the mandible has been completed at this time.

It should be recalled that in the growing boys, the parameters of bone formation were higher on the mesial side than on the distal side in cases of anterior growth rotation and higher on the distal side in posterior growth rotation. The opposite was observed for parameters of bone resorption.

3. In young adult male patients, the alveolar bone turnover rate increase was significant only after three weeks of orthodontic treatment.

Table 7. Continued.

Mesial Side: Alveolar Bone Resorption

β-glucuronidase activity (F.u.)

Season	Inclination	*N*	Median	Range	Multiple comparisons[1] II	III	IV
I. Spring	Anterior	35	25.98	5.74–49.35	**	***	***
II.	Posterior	35	16.12	4.99–49.70		NS	**
III. Autumn	Anterior	35	12.31	2.22–25.92			NS
IV.	Posterior	35	11.61	-0.28–40.94			

T = 19.752 with 3 degrees of freedom
Approximation by χ^2 distribution: p = 0.0002

Acid phenylphosphatase activity (e.u.)

Season	Inclination	*N*	Median	Range	Multiple comparisons[1] II	III	IV
I. Spring	Anterior	35	11.65	2.21–23.29	NS	*	***
II.	Posterior	35	7.99	0.35–22.66		NS	*
III. Autumn	Anterior	35	5.29	1.87–19.64			NS
IV.	Posterior	35	6.19	0.34–22.53			

T = 13.762 with 3 degrees of freedom
Approximation by χ^2 distribution: p = 0.0032

[1]Kruskal-Wallis test: p is the probability that the statement "The effects of a light intermittent mesially-directed force on bone formation will vary according to the mandible inclination and the season" is wrong.

In growing boys, the results were already significant after ten days of orthodontic treatment.

4. In young adult male patients and in growing boys, intermittent orthodontic forces were more effective in producing an increase in the alveolar bone turnover rate than were continuous forces. Light and intermittent forces had a less deleterious effect on the periodontal tissue and on local circulation and allowed for a greater local blood supply on mononuclear bone resorptive and bone forming cell precursors of extrinsic origin.

5. There appears to be a good correlation between a therapeutically-induced increase in alveolar bone turnover rate and the clinical effectiveness of Edgewise treatment.

Table 8. Clinical effectiveness of Edgewise treatment (estimated one year after the onset of treatment) and alveolar bone turnover rate.

Alkaline phenylphosphatase activity (e.u.)

Effectiveness	Anterior *N*	Anterior Median	Anterior Range	Posterior *N*	Posterior Median	Posterior Range
0	10	18.10	16.0-25.60	24	15.25	7.5-23.50
+	43	37.10	16.3-63.60	35	32.85	22.2-67.45
++	14	76.35	37.30-115.30	6	76.75	28.0-89.70
+++	3	74.35	72.01-76.35	5	89.00	70.3-96.00

^{45}Ca uptake (c.p.m.)

Effectiveness	Anterior *N*	Anterior Median	Anterior Range	Posterior *N*	Posterior Median	Posterior Range
0	10	2230.5	1340-2588	24	1509.5	1174-1893
+	43	3259.0	1656-6702	35	2505.0	1598-5583
++	14	7037.0	3284-8907	6	6873.0	2423-7827
+++	3	7608.0	6308-7861	5	7210.0	7127-8053

β-glucuronidase activity (F.u.)

Effectiveness	Anterior *N*	Anterior Median	Anterior Range	Posterior *N*	Posterior Median	Posterior Range
0	10	6.89	5.34-8.73	24	7.10	5.26-8.88
+	43	9.54	6.16-16.92	35	9.08	6.65-22.78
++	14	20.56	12.93-26.66	6	20.95	19.95-21.39
+++	3	22.84	16.70-23.29	5	24.72	22.9-28.49

Acid phenylphosphatase activity (e.u.)

Effectiveness	Anterior *N*	Anterior Median	Anterior Range	Posterior *N*	Posterior Median	Posterior Range
0	10	2.295	2.57-4.04	24	3.18	2.22-3.81
+	43	5.64	2.99-10.49	35	6.02	3.53-7.97
++	14	11.81	8.03-13.76	6	11.31	7.62-12.04
+++	3	10.46	10.06-13.21	5	13.28	12.40-13.52

Anterior = mandible in anterior "inclination"
Posterior = mandible in posterior "inclination"
0: no evidential result
+: poor result
++: suboptimal result
+++: optimal result

REFERENCES

Baron, R. Remaniements de l'os alvéolaire et des fibres desmodontales au cours de la migration physiologique. J. Biol. Buccale. *1:*151-171, 1973.

Baumrind, S. A reconsideration of the propriety of the "pressure-tension' hypothesis. Am. J. Orthod. *55:*12-22, 1969.

Baumrind, S. and D.L. Buck. Rate changes in cell replication and protein synthesis in the periodontal ligament incident to tooth movement. Am. J. Orthod. *57:*109-130, 1970.

Caton, J.G., E.L. DeFuria, A.M. Polson and S. Nyman. Periodontal regeneration via selective cell repopulation. J. Periodontol. *58:*546-552, 1987.

Conover, W.J. *Practical Nonparametric Statistics.* John Wiley and Sons, New York, 1980.

Davidovitch, Z., M.D. Finkelson, S. Steigman, J. Shanfeld, P.C. Montgomery and E. Korostoff. Electric currents, bone remodeling, and orthodontic tooth movement. II. Increase in rate of tooth movement and periodontal cyclic nucleotide levels by combined force and electic current. Am. J. Orthod. 77:33-47, 1980.

Davidovitch, Z., J.L. Shanfeld, P.C. Montgomery, E. Lally, L. Laster, L. Furst, and E. Korostoff. Biochemical mediators of the effects of mechanical forces and electric currents on mineralized tissues. Calcif. Tissue Int. *36:*S86-S97, 1984.

Fruge, J., R. Shaye, and R. Midgett. Histological aspects of tooth movement in hyper-parathyroid dogs. J. Dent. Res. *59(Abstract),* 1980.

Gianelly, A.A. Force induced changes in the vascularity in the periodontal ligament. Am. J. Orthod. *55:*5-11, 1969.

Graber, T.M., D.D.B. Chung and J.T. Aoba. Dentofacial orthopedics versus orthodontics. J.A.D.A. *75:*1145-1166, 1967.

Klinger, E. Etude de l'ostéoclasie alvéolaire par contrainte. Thèse de Doctorat en Sciences Odontologiques, Paris V, 1971.

Kurihara, S. An electronmicroscopic observation on cells found in bone resorption area incident to experimental tooth movement. Bull. Tokyo Med. Dent. Univ. *24:*103-123, 1977.

Kvam, E. A study of the cell-free zone following experimental tooth movement in the rat. Trans. Eur. Orthod. Soc. *45:*419-434, 1970.

Kvam, E. Cellular dynamics on the pressure side of the rate periodontium following experimental tooth movement. Scand. J. Dent. Res. *80:*369-383, 1972.

Lemoine, C. and A. Petrovic. Le marquage à la tetracycline dans les expériences de transplantation dentaire et d'orthodontie chez le rat blanc. Rev. Fr. d'Odonto-stomatol. *9:*1191-1198, 1969.

Lemoine, C., A. Petrovic and J. Stutzmann. Inflammatory process of the rat maxilla after molar autotransplantation. J. Dent. Res. *49:*1175, 1970.

Lilja, E., S. Lindskog and L. Hammarstrom. Histochemistry of enzymes associated with tissue degradation incident to orthodontic tooth movement. Am. J. Orthod. *83:*62-74, 1983.

Macapanpan, L.C., J.P. Weinmann and A.G. Brodie. Early tissue changes following tooth movement in rats. Angle Orthod. *24:*79-95, 1954.

Markostamos, K. Contribution à l'etude des réactions de l'os alvéolaire au cours du déplacement orthodontique expérimental. Thèse de Doctorat en Sciences Odontologiques, Paris V, 1974.

Markostamos, K. and R. Baron. Etude quantitative de l'ostéoclasie sur la paroi alvéolaire au cours de l'orthodontie expérimentale chez le rat. L'Orthod. Fr. *44:*245-258, 1973.

Melsen, B. Tissue reaction following application of extrusive and intrusive forces to teeth in adult monkeys. Am. J. Orthod. *89:*469-475, 1986.

Reitan, K. Continuous bodily tooth movement and histological significance. Acta Odontol. Scand. *7:*115-144, 1947.

Reitan, K. The initial tissue reaction incident to orthodontic tooth movement as related to the influence of function. Acta Odontol. Scand. Suppl. *6:*1-240, 1951.

Reitan, K. Tissue behavior during orthodontic tooth movement. Am. J. Orthod. *46:*881-900, 1960.

Reitan, K. Effects of force magnitude and direction of tooth movement on different alveolar bone types. Angle Orthod. *34:*244-255, 1964.

Reitan, K. Initial tissue behavior during apical root resorption. Angle Orthod. *44:*68-82, 1974.

Roberts, W.E. and D.C. Chase. Kinetics of cell proliferation and migration associated with orthodontically induced osteogenesis. J. Dent. Res. *60:*174-181, 1981.

Rygh, P. Ultrastructural vascular changes in pressure zones of rat molar periodontium incident to orthodontic tooth movement. Scand. J. Dent. Res. *80:*307-321, 1972.

Rygh, P. Ultrastructural changes in pressure zones of human periodontium incident to orthodontic tooth movement. Acta Odont. Scand. *31:*109-122, 1973.

Rygh, P. Elimination of hyalinized periodontal tissues associated with orthodontic tooth movement. Scand. J. Dent. Res. 82:57-73, 1974.

Rygh, P. Periodontal responses to orthodontic forces. In: *Malocclusion and the Periodontium.* J.A. McNamara, Jr. and K.A. Ribbens (Eds.), Monograph 15, Craniofacial Growth Series, Center for Human Growth and Development, The University of Michigan, Ann Arbor, 1984.

Rygh, P. Periodontal response to tooth-moving force: Is trauma necessary? In: *Orthodontics: State of the Art, Essence of the Science.* L.W. Graber (Ed.), C.V. Mosby Co., St. Louis, 1986.

Rygh, P., K. Bowling, L. Howlandsdal and S. Williams. Activation of the vascular system: A main mediator of periodontal fiber remodeling in orthodontic tooth movement. Am. J. Orthod. *89:*453-468, 1986.

Rygh, P., K. Bowling, L. Howlandsdal and S. Williams. Activation of the vascular system: Another main mediator of periodontal fiber remodeling in orthodontic tooth movement (in preparation).

Rygh, P. and K. Selvig. Erythrocytic crystallization in rat molar periodontium incident to orthodontic tooth movement. Scand. J. Dent. Res. *80:*62-73, 1973.

Shanfeld, J., J.L. Jones, L. Laster and Z. Davidovitch. Biochemical aspects of orthodontic tooth movement. I. Cyclic nucleotide and prostaglandin concentrations in tissues surrounding orthodontically treated teeth in vivo. Am. J. Orthod. Dentofac. Orthop. *90:*139-148, 1986.

Siegel, S. *Nonparametric Statistics for the Behavioral Sciences.* International Student Edition, McGraw-Hill, 1956.

Stark, T.M. and P.M. Sinclair. Effect of pulsed electromagnetic fields on orthodontic tooth movement. Am. J. Orthod. Dentofac. Orthop. *91:*91-104, 1987.

Stein, G. and J. Weinmann. Die physiologische Wanderung der Zahne. Z. Stomatol. *23:*733-744, 1925.

Storey, E. Bone changes associated with tooth movement. A histological study of the effect of force for varying duration in the rabbit, guinea pig and rat. Aust. Dent. J. *59:*209-219, 1955.

Stutzmann, J. and A. Petrovic. Human alveolar bone turn-over rate. A quantitative study of spontaneous and therapeutically-induced variations. In: *Malocclusion and the Periodontium.* J.A. McNamara, Jr. and K.A. Ribbens (Eds.), Craniofacial Growth Series, Center for Human Growth and Development, University of Michigan, Ann Arbor, 1984.

Stutzmann, J. and A. Petrovic. Spontaneous and therapeutically-induced variations of the human alveolar bone turn-over rate. A quantitative study. Nova Acta Leopoldina NF 58, *262:*77-91, 1986.

Stutzmann, J., A. Petrovic and R. Shaye. Analyse en culture organotypique de la vitesse de formation-résorption de l'os alvéolaire humain prélevé avant et pendant un traitement comprenant le déplacement des dents: Nouvelle voie d'approche en recherche orthodontique. L'Orthod. Fr. *50:*399-419, 1979.

Stutzmann, J., A. Petrovic and R. Shaye. Analyse der Resorptionsbildungsgeschwindigkeit des menschlichen Alveolarknochens, in organotypischer Kultur, entnomen vor und waehrend der Durchführung einer Zahnbewegung. Ein neuer Anblick in der orthodontischer Forschung. Fortschr. Kieferorth. *41:*236-250, 1980.

Yamasaki, K., Y. Shibata, S. Imai, Y. Tani, Y. Shibasaki and T. Fukuhara. Clinical application of prostaglandin E (PGE_1) upon orthodontic tooth movement. Am. J. Orthod. *85:*508-518, 1984.